ENCYCLOPEDIA OF MEDICINAL FOODS

Combines in one handy volume information on the nutritive value of foods, what foods are best for treating various ailments and how to prepare foods to best advantage.

ENCYCLOPEDIA OF MEDICINAL FOODS

by
Joseph M. Kadans N.D., Ph.D.

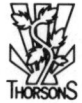

THORSONS PUBLISHERS LIMITED
Wellingborough, Northamptonshire

First published in the United Kingdom 1979

*Original American edition published as 'Encyclopedia of Fruits,
Vegetables, Nuts and Seeds for Healthful Living'
by Parker Publishing Company, Inc., West Nyack, New York.*

ISBN 0 7225 0580 9 (paperback)
ISBN 0 7225 0582 5 (hardback)

Printed and bound in Great Britain by
Biddles Ltd., Guildford, Surrey

Dedicated to my darling wife, Adele, without whose devotion, patience and forbearing this work would never have been completed.

WHAT THIS BOOK CAN DO FOR YOU

Much has been said and written about the health-building values of various foods and especially about fruits, vegetables, nuts and seeds. However, there has not been a modern single-volume home encyclopedia published concerning specific health values of these foods. This book takes up each important food in each classification as above in alphabetical order, describes their nutritive and health values, explains what unhealthy conditions they may probably help and offers suggestions on preparing these health foods as "Nature's Medicines." It is a generally accepted fact that food can be your best medicine.

There is a section that explains the various nutritive factors—the vitamins and minerals in each food—and also describes the practical functions of the digestive processes such as enzymes, acid-alkaline balance, and other vital information. It sets out recommended daily allowances, minimum daily requirements and explanations of calories, proteins, amino acids, lecithin, niacin etc. Many other questions relative to healthful nutrition and dietetics are also answered.

Finally, there is the *Symptomatic-Locator Index*. If you have a symptom of ill health or impending bad health, the index will locate and indicate the food remedy for your consideration.

Let us assume that someone has stomach cramps. By looking through the index for "Stomach cramps, help for," one can learn just what foods are recommended for persons with this condition, together with instructions for preparation of the foods. Thus, the index can be a convenient guide for dieticians in hospitals and for physicians who need to prescribe for their patients the kind of diet best suited for the particular ailment. Likewise, people who are themselves ill and who prefer to help themselves will be able to rely upon this exhaustive compilation of data on nutrition. Better yet, those who want to stay well and avoid illness would do well to note the rules of diet set forth in this volume.

Incidentally, a fringe benefit is the example you may be setting for your young and impressionable children. In these days when so many young people become addicted to drugs, some experts say that these young people have learned from their parents to "take pills for all problems." By avoiding the pill bottles and using natural foods containing nature's medicines, the pill habit can be broken. Remember, too, that the pills and drugs might not contain the enzymes and other factors needed by the body for good health.

In conditions where heavy concentrations of vitamins or minerals are needed, it would pay to invest in a good fruit and vegetable juicer and/or blender to allow easier digestion and assimilation of the various food items. However, this is optional with the reader.

This book is of unique value because of problems regarding nutrition that plague us all. Who has not read or heard that some particular food item is good, but to read or hear later that it was bad for you? There is just too much confusion for the average person in the nutrition field, and after many years of research and study of the leading authorities in the nutrition field, this encyclopedia, in an organized way, is a "breakthrough" for simple answers without confusion.

The book also serves the man or woman who lives alone and who wants to know what to eat to maintain good health or to help recover it. It is also meant for the home-maker, who purchases food for the family and who wants her family to have nourishing food of high quality and delicious taste, as well as being economical and well-prepared.

This encyclopedia may be called the "Natural Food Bible" as it deals with the natural foods such as existed at the time of the Bible to the present day, the natural fruits, vegetables, nuts and seeds. This convenient reference book, together with its exclusive index, has been designed to be a complete source of information not only with regard to the particular values of particular foods, but also filling the gap for providing authoritative explanations of various aspects of the digestive processes for better health.

Thus, there are many unique features not found in any other compilation of healthful food data. While there are books that give nutritive values of foods, and there are books that advise what foods are best for treating various ailments, depending upon the vitamins and minerals in the foods, and there are books that tell how to prepare foods, there has been no book known to combine all three of these important requirements in one.

In addition, all of the important vitamins and minerals are explained in a simple manner that anyone can understand. This will be of great help in dispelling the confusion and misunderstanding that is so common today. For example, some people will avoid eating acid-forming foods for fear of acidosis, whereas the section explaining digestive terms points out that acid-forming foods as well as alkaline-forming foods are both vital for a healthy body.

The outstanding unique and exclusive feature is the *Symptomatic-Locator Index* for this treasury of food information. If you want to locate any information about a food, see this unique index for a reference to the page where the information is located. If you know of some symptom of disease and you want to know what food, vitamin, mineral, or other substance is indicated for relief of the symptom, just look up the symptom in the index and you will obtain both a reference to the food or foods or other substance where the symptom is mentioned, and the page number. This gives you instant reference and guidance regarding matters of food affecting your health.

It will pay you to consult the food-preparation section of this encyclopedia. In this section, there will be found numerous innovations in food preparation so as to preserve, whenever possible, the inherent goodness of each food, protecting the vitamins from destruction in the cooking processes in many cases and at the same time preserving the valuable enzymes and other factors from being boiled to destruction and killing their subtle health values. It is emphasized, however, that this is not just another raw-food cooking section.

I am confident that your regular use of this book will help you to gain more natural dynamic health and save you money in the process.

Joseph M. Kadans, N.D., Ph.D.

ACKNOWLEDGMENTS

Several pages of bibliography might have been included at the end of the volume as proof of the use of authentic material. In lieu of this, I would like to especially acknowledge the helpfulness of such source materials as:

"The Avitaminoses" by Walter H. Eddy, Ph.D. and Gilbert Dalldorf, M.D. (Williams & Wilkins Company), dealing with the chemical, clinical and pathological aspects of the vitamin deficiency diseases;

"Chemistry of Organic Compounds" by Carl R. Noller, Professor of Chemistry, Stanford University (W. B. Saunders Company);

"Essentials of Biological and Medical Physics" by Ralph W. Stacy, Ph.D., Department of Physiology, Ohio State University, David T. Williams, Ph.D., Physicist, Battelle Memorial Institute, Columbus, Ohio, Ralph E. Worden, M.D., College of Medicine, Ohio State University and Rex O. McMorris, M.D., University of Louisville Medical School (McGraw-Hill Book Company, Inc.);

"Nutrition and Physical Fitness" by L. Jean Bogert, Ph.D., Professor of Food Economics and Nutrition, Kansas State University, George M. Briggs, Ph.D., Chairman and Professor of Nutrition, Department of Nutritional Sciences, University of California at Berkeley, (W. B. Saunders Company);

"Taber's Cyclopedic Medical Dictionary" by Clarence Wilbur Taber (F. A. Davis Company);

"Nutrition In Health and Disease" by Lenna F. Cooper, Sc.D., Edith M. Barber, M.S., Helen S. Mitchell, Ph.D. and Henderika J. Rynbergen, M.S. (J. B. Lippincott Company);

"Biochemistry and Physiology of Nutrition" by Geoffrey H. Bourne, Department of Histology, London Hospital Medical College, London, England and George W. Kidder, Biological Laboratory, Amherst College, Amherst, Massachusetts (Academic Press).

CONTENTS

PART II - ANALYSIS OF NUTRITIVE BENEFITS OF FRUITS, VEGETABLES, NUTS AND SEEDS

PART III - THE SYMPTOMATIC LOCATOR INDEX

PART I
COMPONENTS OF MEDICINES AND HEALING AGENTS IN FOODS LISTED

ADRENOCORTICOTROPIC HORMONE (ACTH)

Explanation. There is a tiny gland at the base of the brain, the pituitary, which secretes hormones. When needed, they are sent into the blood and supplied to the two small glands above the kidneys known as the adrenal glands. The adrenal glands also manufacture adrenaline, a hormone thought to be concerned with maintenance of the tonus of blood vessels and the heart. Deficiencies of vitamins such as Vitamins A, B_2 or E and a deficiency in linoleic acid may limit the production of hormones. In fact, practically all vitamins, especially Vitamin C, are needed by the body for proper functioning of the glands and organs. Pantothenic acid, for example, may cause a marked decrease in the quantity of hormones produced.

Tensions and stresses. When the brain senses danger or where there is any unusual stress such as exercise, the glands produce hormones, cortisone and sex hormones as needed by the various parts of the body to meet the tension or stress demands. Proteins are broken down to form sugar for energy to meet the demands of the muscles or organs requiring attention. The stress causes the heart to beat faster, blood pressure to increase, and fat is drawn from storage centers. Intense stress continuing without pause, such as injuries from a serious automobile accident or other injuries, may exhaust the body reserves and cause serious results, perhaps even death. For example, stomach ulcers may result from the stress taking protein from the stomach walls, depriving the lining of the stomach of the protection it normally enjoys. Likewise, ulcerative colitis may take place in the colon for the same reason. It is no wonder that worried people get ulcers.

Sources of ACTH: The anti-stress factors important for meeting stress demands are found in wheat germ, in the pulp of green leafy vegetables, some yeasts, and soy flour from which the oil has not been removed. For meat eaters, liver and kidneys are highest in these anti-stress substances.

AMINO ACIDS

Value: Amino acids are used in the digestive processes. Tryptophane, cystine, lysine and histidine are necessary for tissue repair and growth. Hydroxyaminobutyric acid, isoleucine, leucine and phenylalanine are other essential amino acids. While amino acids are found largely in proteins, which are transformed into amino acids in the intestines and are found also in the bloodstream, all proteins do not contain all the essential amino acids. The recommended amount of protein for body weight should be one gram of protein for each kilogram (2.2 lb.) of body weight. For a person weighing 100 pounds, there should be a minimum of 50 grams of protein daily. Too often, individuals on fruit or vegetable diets do not get sufficient protein.

Result of deficiency. The body needs a sufficient variety of proteins so that all of the essential amino acids are provided. Where there is a lack of amino acids, the body tissues suffer in their maintenance and upkeep. In addition to physicial weakness, it is difficult for the mind to cope with the mental and emotional stresses and strains of modern living.

Availability. While meat is said to be the most perfect protein, it is sometimes difficult to obtain meat produced from cattle that has not been injected with chemicals to fatten them for the market or cattle fed with clean grains and grass. In many areas, the air has become polluted with atomic fallout that lands in the fields and is ingested by cattle and imbedded into the tissues. While lean meat has a heavy concentration of proteins, such foods as nuts, legumes (such as beans, lentils and peas), eggs and cheese have valuable protein content with ample supplies of amino acids. Yogurt is an ideal protein food and may be considered as a substitute for meat. In addition, it is rich in friendly bacteria which, with the lactic acid in the yogurt, act as an intestinal disinfectant.

ACIDITY AND ALKALINITY

In general: There has been some confusion as to the acidity and alkalinity of various foods and the need for maintaining a balance. The body has a first, second and third line of defense against excessive acidity or alkalinity, as the maintenance of neutrality in the blood and tissues is too vital to the well-being of the body to be left entirely to random selection of foods by the individual.

The three defenses. (1) Buffer substances in the blood and tissues (phosphates and carbonates) take up excessive acid or alkali substances.

(2) When there is excessive alkalinity (base-forming foods or substances), the body uses a reserve acid, carbonic acid, to neutralize the excessive acidity.

(3) When there is excessive acidity (for example, excessive sulfuric and phosphoric acids due to overeating of protein foods), the body uses a reserve of alkaline fluid, ammonia, formed by the kidneys when needed, to neutralize the excessive acidity.

Protein elements. One of the functions of protein is to help maintain the acid-alkaline balance of the blood or of the tissues. The normal condition should be a neutral balance or very slightly alkaline, and as proteins are able to unite with either acid or alkaline substances, an ample supply of protein will aid the body in maintaining a proper balance.

Mineral elements. Mineral elements also participate in regulating the acid-alkaline balance. Just as protein elements unite with either acid or alkaline substances, some of the mineral elements give rise in metabolism to acidic and others to alkaline substances. The two substances can then be paired off together to form neutral substances called salts. The principal acid-forming mineral elements are sulfur, phosphorus and chlorine, and the principal alkaline (base-forming) elements are sodium, potassium, calcium, magnesium and iron.

Food balance. It is desirable to ingest an approximate equal amount of both acid-forming and alkaline-forming food. In general, the acid-forming foods are usually the high-protein foods, often containing sulfur and phosphorus. Fruits and vegetables are mainly alkaline-forming, as they contain large quantities of alkaline elements either as inorganic salts or as salts of organic acids that can be burned in the body. The ingestion of ample quantities of fruits and vegetables also supplies vitamins and fiber as well as alkaline-forming elements, and it is the combination of all these factors that makes them so beneficial.

BLOOD COUNTS

In general: Blood is the fluid that circulates in the veins, arteries, heart and capillaries. It is the principal medium by which the tissues of the body are nourished and relieved of waste or effete matter. The blood is mainly a plasma in which corpuscles are suspended. There are red and white corpuscles. When observed under a microscope, a red corpuscle resembles a tiny doughnut in shape. The white corpuscles or leucocytes appear as tiny speckled balls.

Number: In a cubic millimeter of human blood, there are normally about 5,000,000 red corpuscles and from 5,000 to 7,000 white corpuscles. The average person of average weight and height has five quarts of blood and for this amount of blood, it would be necessary to have about thirty-five trillion red blood cells floating around. Good red blood should score 100 on the hemoglobin scale, which would be 15.6 grams in 100 cc. (half a cup) of blood. The national average blood count is from 70 to 85, which borders on anemia. Anyone having a blood count below 60 definitely has anemia. When the blood count drops to 35 or lower, it is necessary to have a blood transfusion to add red corpuscles to the blood.

CALORIES

In the field of dietetics, a calorie is the unit of measurement of heat or energy production. Just as an automobile will not run without gasoline, so will the human body not run without food containing calories. A diet of food rich with calories will supply lots of energy but will also increase the body weight, as calorie-rich foods are usually amply supplied with fat. To reduce weight, foods with fat must be avoided and the body will thereupon reach out for supplies of fat stored in the body in order to meet the needs of the body for calories to support energy-expending activities.

Restriction to a 1,200 calorie diet is the customary remedy of physicians for persons wishing to reduce. The diet should include sufficient bulk to prevent hunger pangs, enough protein for the usual functioning of the body (not less than 50 grams), sufficient carbohydrates (about 125 grams), and adequate supplies of minerals and vitamins.

A smaller calorie ration of approximately 900 calories daily may be necessary for stubborn obesity cases. However, it must be noted that even though the body may draw from stored fat supplies to cope with the energy demands of the body, there may not be an immediate weight loss because of replacement of the fat by water.

However, it is not too long before the water also leaves the body and the weight reduction becomes noticeable.

The caloric value of fruits is comparatively low. The chief caloric value of fruits is from the carbohydrate values of fruits, usually in the form of sugar. While dried fruits have high caloric value when eaten as such, most people take the dried fruits and soak them in water, hot or cold, to soften them. After their water content is restored, the caloric value is similar to the fruit in its original form. Canned and frozen fruits have higher caloric values because of the sugar used in preparation. The high fat content of the avocado, pear and the olive gives these fruits a high caloric value.

With the exception of soybeans, the fat content of vegetables is quite low, and in order to insure an adequate supply of vitamins and minerals it is necessary to ingest an abundant supply of vegetables in the diet. The dry legumes, such as beans, are high in calories because they are high in carbohydrates as well as in protein. Potatoes have many calories due to the high starch content while other vegetables, such as beets and sweet potatoes, have high caloric values because they are quite rich in sugar.

A good reason for eating lots of vegetables is that almost all vegetables have nondigestible cellulose and hemicellulose, which aids in peristalsis or movement of waste through the intestines.

Vegetables may look alike and may even taste alike, but due to differences in the type of soil, the methods of fertilizing, and the care taken during growth, packing and transportation to market, they may be different with regard not only to caloric value but also in the contents of vitamins and minerals.

Nuts are high in caloric value, from peanut butter to coconuts. Calories range from approximately 200 calories per one hundred grams to over 700 calories per 100 grams for filberts, hickory nuts, raw pecans and English walnuts. Almost equal in calorie value are unblanched almonds, shelled Brazil nuts, shredded coconut, peanuts and pistachios. Nuts that are chopped or ground are more easily digested. For vegetarians, nuts are a necessary part of the diet, as there are relatively few proteins in vegetables alone

CARBOHYDRATES

Value. Carbohydrates provide energy, heat and a small amount is stored in the liver as glycogen for future use. Excess carbohydrates are stored in the body as fat. Insulin, secreted by the pancreas, is needed for the utilization of carbohydrates by the body. Carbohydrates are classified as starches, sugars, glycogen, gums, and cellulose, the fiber of plants and vegetable cells. The undigested cellulose furnishes the bulk often necessary for efficient and normal peristaltic action of the intestines. All carbohydrates, other than the cellulose, must be transformed to glucose before they can be utilized by the body. Excessive carbohydrates in the diet is the chief cause of overweight.

Results of deficiency. The glucose manufactured by the body and then transported by the blood to the tissues gives energy to the muscles. Insufficient carbohydrates will make a person feel tired because of this lack of glucose. When there is an inadequate supply, the liver releases glucose manufactured from the glycogen in the liver with the help of the insulin from the pancreas. Just as constant withdrawals of funds from a limited bank account will soon deplete the account, so will withdrawals of glucose from the liver, which is really a reserve supply, deplete the supply of glycogen, from which the glucose is made. This may also over-work the pancreas, due to the function of the pancreas in supplying insulin for the manufacture of the glucose. Consequently, a breakdown of the pancreas may lead to diabetes.

A lack of carbohydrates will interfere with the normal metabolism of other foodstuffs. The condition known as acidosis may result from insufficient carbohydrates, as without carbohydrates there is incomplete oxidation of fatty acids and they become toxic to the body. Fatty acids do not oxidize as readily as do sugars in the body, and carbohydrates help to obtain a good oxidation.

Additionally, a deficiency in carbohydrates and glucose interferes with milk production in the female as the mammary glands, through enzyme action, manufacture lactose from the blood glucose. (Lactose is milk sugar.)

Availability. Carbohydrates are present in heaviest quantities from foods such as candy bars, cooked sweet potatoes, cookies, ice cream, breads and rolls, bananas, peas, beans, potatoes, corn, and parsnips. It should hardly be necessary to add that such sweets as candy bars, cookies and ice cream should be avoided except on special occasions, when slight deviations from good food may be tolerated. Of course, bread and rolls should be avoided because of the heavy starch content in the flour and the digestive difficulties that often follow.

CARBOHYDRATES-INOSITOL

Value. This carbohydrate is deemed to be essential for good nutrition. The precise function is uncertain but reports indicate that there is some association with the metabolism or transport of fat, it having the capacity of preventing the accumulation of fat in the liver. When combined with Vitamin E, it is said to help in cases of muscular dystrophy.

Results of deficiency. Studies by nutritionists indicate that a deficiency of inositol may cause coronary heart attacks and accumulations of fat in the liver, causing faulty liver functioning. A fatty liver is common in diabetes and thus it may be assumed that a deficiency of inositol is a contributing factor in connection with that disease. A shortage of inositol is also reported to interfere with the adequate production of lecithin, necessary for the control of fat in the blood. In experiments with animals, it has been found that a lack of inositol will result in a complete loss of hair. Based upon reports of investigators, it would be desirable to include at least 1000 mg. of inositol daily to avoid a deficiency of this nutrient.

Availability. The richest natural sources are yeast, wheat germ, and the soybean. In animal tissues, the largest amounts are found in the liver and kidney, as well as in skeletal and heart muscle. In plants, it is present in abundance in the leaves.

ENZYMES

An enzyme is a complex chemical substance produced by animals and plants and is found particularly in the digestive juices. Enzymes act upon other substances and cause them to split up into simpler substances. The enzyme, as a catalytic agent, induces chemical changes in other substances but remains unchanged itself. The chemist explains this action by stating that the enzyme, when combining with other substances, produces a compound too unstable to exist under the conditions. The compound then immediately breaks up.

There are at least a dozen significant digestive enzymes in the secretions of the digestive juices. They aid in digesting fats, proteins and carbohydrates. The saliva contains an enzyme which acts on starch to convert it into sugar. When the food enters the stomach, it is further disintegrated or broken up by the enzymes in the stomach.

Pepsin and hydrochloric acid act to break down protein in the stomach. Milk entering the stomach is coagulated by the action of the hydrochloric acid, pepsin, and other substances such as rennin. There is both a mechanical and chemical action in the stomach that requires about four hours to function.

Many of the enzymes and the specific actions involved can be determined by the name assigned to the enzyme. For example, when the enzyme ends with the letters "ase" it means that the enzyme is a hydrolytic enzyme. This type of enzyme causes the elimination of water, the word "hydro" being, of course, a reference to water. During the process of digestion, water taken into the body loses its identity as water but becomes another substance because of the enzymes contacted by it. This happens with all food taken into the body. Enzymes break down the food. Some of the hydrolytic enzymes are lipases, which specialize in splitting fats; amylases, which split starches; and proteases, the enzymes that split proteins.

Each enzyme can act only upon a particular substance at exactly the right temperature, acidity, alkalinity, or other conditions. The body manufactures enzymes out of food, water and air, these being the only ingredients available. Each enzyme is specific; that is, each acts only on a certain type of substance and brings about only one special chemical reaction.

There are certain enzymes in the mouth, others in the stomach, and still others in the small intestine. Each digestive enzyme has a degree of acidity or alkalinity (known as the optimum reaction) at which it works best. Also, there is a range of reaction, so that if the alkalinity is too high or too low or the acidity too high or too low the enzyme will not function. The same applies to the temperature, which must be just right, and in addition there must be good surface contact with the substance acted upon, which is called the substrate. Also, for best or optimum results, the products of digestion must be continuously removed by absorption.

Because enzymes are living cells, they are sensitive to heat and cold. Consequently, boiling temperatures will destroy them and cold temperatures will suspend their activity. The enzymes that digest food work best at the temperature of the body. When enzymes ordinarily present in food are destroyed by cooking, the body is required to manufacture more enzymes. A large share of enzyme production is borne by the pancreas, and it is theorized that if people ate more uncooked foods and thus absorbed natural enzymes into the bodily system, the pancreas would not be overworked and it would not be necessary for the pancreas to produce so much pancreatic juice. Malfunction of the pancreas, due to overwork, upsets the digestion of proteins, fats and other substances.

One of the internal secretions of the pancreas is insulin, which controls carbohydrates An inability of the body to properly utilize carbohydrates and fats is characterized as diabetes mellitus. This inability causes blood sugar to rise to abnormal heights, and it then passes into the urine. When this happens, the sugar loss becomes so large that the body supply of sugar falls below normal and the condition known as hypoglycemia is the result.

There is another theory supporting the belief that men and women would live to a really ripe old age if they conserved their enzyme supply in the body. It is claimed that when men lived on fruits, nuts, berries, raw meat and unheated natural milk, without destruction of the enzymes in food, their bodies would not be worn out so soon by producing more and more enzymes necessary to digest foods deprived of enzymes due to destruction by boiling or other processing. There are medical histories indicating that the pancreas becomes larger as a person eats more and more cooked starches.

In addition to the manufacture of enzymes in the salivary glands and the pancreas, glands located in the membrane lining of the stomach secrete gastric juices. Glands in the intestinal walls produce enzymes that act to complete the digestion of certain carbohydrates into simple sugars and perform other important functions.

In any discussion of enzymes, we must not forget the liver, the chief function of which is to aid digestion. It mainly secretes bile, which in turn stimulates other secretions, promotes peristalsis and checks bacterial action. Bile salts are needed for the digestion of fats. The liver also stores carbohydrates for future conversion into sugar for energy when needed. The carbohydrates are stored in the liver in the form of glycogen. As an enzyme, it is known as glycogenase and its end product is dextrose, a simple sugar formed from the action of acids on starches. Dextrose also occurs naturally in the juices of plants and the body fluids of animals.

There is no doubt that many cases of overweight (the term "obesity" is not used unless the individual is from 20 to 30 percent over the average weight for his age and height) are due to bodily craving for food and nutrients. Perhaps if more care would be taken to partake of natural foods such as fruits, vegetables, nuts, and seeds, the body would obtain its needed share of enzymes and the craving for excessive amounts of food would disappear. It must be remembered that enzymes not only digest food but they also convert sugars into energy, so that we may move about. Our organs and tissues need the molecules produced by enzymes for growth or for replacement. In addition, enzymes generate more enzymes.

The overweight condition can easily lead to heart disease, as the heart is overburdened by the strain of carrying unnecessary weight. Overeating also places excessive strain upon the liver, spleen, gall-bladder, kidneys and other organs of the body, due to the effort involved in processing all of the food taken into the body unnecessarily in order to meet the bodily needs for the enzymes.

Too little is known about cancer to attribute the lack of enzymes as a causative factor in the production of cancer. However, it would not be surprising, as research continues, to learn that cancer does not attack persons partaking of natural foods and thus acquiring an ample amount of natural enzymes needed by the body.

FATS

When broken into basic chemical elements, fat is composed of carbon, hydrogen, and a small proportion of oxygen. Each gram of fat yields nine calories of heat or energy.

Any type of fat is composed of four molecules, of which three are fatty acids and one molecule is glycerol. Some fatty acids have carbon atoms which will not accept additional hydrogen, and these are called saturated fatty acids. When hydrogen can be added to a fatty acid group, such a group is called mono-unsaturated or poly-unsaturated, depending upon whether hydrogen can be added at one or more of the links in the chain of carbon.

Most food contains a mixture of both saturated and unsaturated fatty acids and in order to simplify the classification of foods, the fat in food is called saturated if there are more saturated fatty acids than unsaturated and it is called unsaturated if there is a lesser amount of saturated fatty acids.

The saturated fatty acids contain stearic acid, which is found in such food fats as beef and mutton, as well as other animal fats, including the milk of cows. It is also found in some vegetable fats. When there are high proportions of saturated fatty acids, the fat is usually in a solid state; otherwise, when low in saturated fatty acids, it is usually in a liquid state.

Oleic acid is an oil compound consisting of 18 parts carbon, 34 parts hydrogen and two parts oxygen, and is found in most mixed oils and fats. It is part of the mono-unsaturated fatty acid group and is contained in olive oil, peanut oil and other food fats.

The poly-unsaturated fats are found in soybean, corn, cottonseed, and other vegetable oils. This group of fats contains linoleic acid, a thin, yellow, oil compound consisting of eighteen parts carbon, 32 parts hydrogen and two parts oxygen.

In stearic acid, found in saturated fatty acids, the amount of carbon (18) is the same as in oleic acid and linoleic acid; however, the hydrogen portion is thirty-six parts as compared with the 34 parts of oleic acid and the 32 parts of linoleic acid. As in the other acids, stearic acid contains only two parts of oxygen.

Because of the small amount of oxygen in the various fatty acids, fats require a considerable amount of oxygen in the oxidizing processes of the body.

An important hormone, cholecystokinin, is produced as a result of digestion of fats in the small intestine. This hormone stimulates the gallbladder to send bile into the small intestine and it is the bile that emulsifies or degenerates the fat, breaking it into tiny globules or particles. An enzyme juice from the pancreas, known as pancreatic lipase, splits fatty compounds into fatty acids and glycerol, another name for glycerin. Glycerin is a triatomic alcohol formed as a result of decomposition of natural fats by alkalis.

While excessive fat deposits in the body produce extra burdens on the heart and generally interfere with the functioning of many organs of the body, it must be recognized that some fat is needed. A gram of fat contributes more than twice as much energy as a gram of protein or of carbohydrate, namely, nine calories. Some additional fat deposits present in the body make the fat available for use as energy or heat at all times. Without the fat reserve supply, individuals would need to eat more often for the necessary constant supply of energy needed by the body.

Fatty tissue provides an insulation beneath the skin and thus helps to maintain the required body temperature. Fat also serves as a cushion for protection against accidental bruises, contusions or traumatic injuries near vital organs of the body such as the kidneys or vertebrae of the spine. In addition, an ample supply of fatty tissue provides a feeling of fullness and staves off hunger pangs for a considerable period of time. Fatty foods also contribute a flavor and taste to the diet that enhances the enjoyment of food.

Good health requires that the body have the benefit of certain essential fatty acids. Linoleic acid, for example, cannot be manufactured by the body, but it is necessary for normal growth and especially for a healthy skin. Another fatty acid, arachic acid, is found in butter and other substances, but when linoleic acid is present the body can change linoleic acid to arachic acid when it is needed. Another fatty acid, important to brain and nerve tissue, is the group of fatty acids known as phospholipids, containing phosphorus and nitrogen. They assist in the absorption of fat into the blood circulation.

According to studies of eating habits, the fat intake of the average individual in the United States is about forty percent of all calories consumed. While some health authorities recommend that the fat intake be limited to 20 or 25 percent of the total intake of calories, there are other areas of the world, such as Asia and Africa, where the fat intake is as little as 10 percent of the total intake and the people seem to be in good health. At the other extreme, the Eskimo's diet will include a very large percentage of fat intake without apparent harmful effect.

The most sensible and reasonable plan is to balance the fat intake with the needs of the body. Health authorities recommend that the minimum fat intake be at least 25 to 50 grams daily, with a maximum intake of 100 grams daily.

Experimental studies with animals have indicated that where fat is excluded from the diet scaly skin lesions develop, the kidneys become deranged, bleeding takes place from the mucous membrane of the urinary passages (hematuria), growth is retarded, males become sterile, females produce poor litters, nursing mothers do not give adequate milk, and the deficiency finally results in death.

In experiments with humans, excellent results were obtained in certain limited areas of experimentation. For example, in cases of infantile eczema, it was found that corn oil or lard in the diet restored the skin to normalcy.

 Rancid fat, resulting from oxidation due to staleness or excessive heat as occurring in fry-pans, causes considerable harm to the body. Rancid fat destroys Vitamins A and E and damages some of the B vitamins. Experiments with animals by feeding them rancid fat produced deficiency diseases of the type that would occur in the event of Vitamin A or E deficiencies. Further study with humans is badly needed to ascertain the precise effect of intake of rancid fat.

FOLIC ACID

Value. Folic acid has been recognized as one of the B vitamins necessary for good nutrition. Its chemical formula is $C_{19}H_{19}N_7O_6$

and it is slightly soluble in water and easily oxidized in acid and sun light. It helps in the growth of a healthy blood system and aids the intestinal tract to stay healthy. It has been indicated that up to three milligrams daily would be an adequate amount. The bacteria in the intestines will ordinarily work to combine or synthesize various elements together to form folic acid.

Results of deficiency. A deficiency of this B vitamin may have serious results for the expectant mother. The condition of a congenital fissure or split in the roof of the mouth, known as cleft palate, may be the result of a deficiency in folic acid substance. Also, although it is not certain, this deficiency may contribute to other conditions of the newborn child such as horseshoe kidneys (union of the kidneys at the lower ends), hydrocephalus (fluid within the cranium), harelip, and heart and brain defects.

Anemia is one of the conditions that may result from a deficiency in folic acid. Individuals taking such drugs as aminopterin, streptomycin and the sulfa drugs must be warned that these drugs destroy folic acid.

The condition known as sprue, where there is a sore mouth, indigestion and diarrhea, may also result from the lack of folic acid. There may also result a shortage of the large red blood corpuscles, the condition known as megaloblastic anemia.

Availability. It is found abundantly in spinach, watercress, and the greens of mustard, beet turnips, parsley, carrots, broccoli, and generally in almost all green leaves of vegetables and herbs. It is also found in mushrooms, soybeans and wheat germ. For non-vegetarians, it is also found in liver and milk.

LECITHIN

Value. Lecithin is one of the derivatives of glycerin and is of value for cases of malnutrition, rickets, anemia, diabetes and tuberculosis. It is known as a phospholipid and is formed by the union of one molecule of glycerol, two molecules of fatty acid and one molecule each of phosphoric acid and choline, a nitrogenous base. Lecithin helps in the structural support of all cells, especially of the brain and nerves. It is important in preventing and correcting atherosclerosis, causing cholesterol and neutral fats to be broken into microscopic particles so they can be more easily utilized by the tissues. Usually one or two tablespoons daily will keep the fat in the blood at normal levels. It is also of value in relieving the angina pectoris pain in the region of the heart to the left shoulder and arm.

Results of deficiency. Heart disease resulting from atherosclerosis (degeneration of walls of the arteries) due to lack of sufficient lecithin is a common result. While the body will usually produce lecithin to cope with a meal that is high in fat or excessive in calories, with a condition of atherosclerosis, gradually built up over a period of time, the fat particles will often be unable to pass through the arterial walls and consequently remain in the arteries. A vicious circle develops and as more fatty deposits form on the arterial walls, the more difficult it is for the fat molecules to pass through the tiny capillaries into the tissue for utilization as energy.

Availability. Lecithin occurs in all unrefined foods containing oil. Paint manufacturers use vegetable oil, but because lecithin makes the paint smear it is separated from the vegetable oil and is sold as a side-product in granular form for adding to foods. It is widely used commercially as an emulsifying agent in the candy and baking industries, as well as in heavy industries where oil must be broken down into tiny particles. When added to gravies, the fat seems to literally disappear. It is also available from eggs, liver, nuts, wheat and soy oil.

LINOLEIC ACID

Value. This is a thin, yellow, oily compound, $C_{18}H_{22}O_2$, found in various drying oils such as linseed, poppy and hemp. Individuals with excessively high blood cholesterol may usually reduce the cholesterol level by ingesting vegetable oils rich in linoleic acid. The more solid fats eaten, the more need for linoleic acid. In addition to linoleic acid, there are two other fatty acids needed before cholesterol and saturated fats can be utilized, namely linolenic acid and arachic acid, a crystalline fatty compound contained in butter and other substances. Linolenic acid is a component of linseed and soybean oils. Linoleic or linolenic acid must be supplied by fats ingested into the body to insure a healthy condition of the skin. Linoleic, linolenic and arachic or arachadonic fatty acids are of the poly-unsaturated variety.

Result of deficiency. Any deficiency results in a tendency toward build-up of crust in arteries, the condition known as arteriosclerosis, especially when the intake of solid fats is high. Linoleic acid is a nutrient that utilizes the natural saturated fats of the body, thus preventing fat build-ups throughout the body tissues. One indication of a high cholesterol level in the blood is the appearance of yellow fatty accumulations in the skin around the eyes. Sometimes these fat accumulations may appear in other parts of the body, such as around the breasts or in the abdominal and pelvic area.

Availability. Many vegetable oils are rich in linoleic acid, such as safflower oil, sunflower-seed oil, sesame-seed oil, walnut oil and soy oil. Linoleic acid is also found in corn oil, peanut oil, cottonseed oil, and a smaller amount in olive oil. Human milk and commercially prepared formulas usually provide sufficient linoleic acid, but formulas involving the use of evaporated milk barely meet the minimum requirements. When there is doubt as to providing a sufficient amount, the diet of infants could be supplemented by feeding the infant whole grain cereals.

MINERALS–CALCIUM

Value. Calcium helps to build and maintain bones and teeth, helps to heal wounds, offsets the effect of acid, and heals wounds. It has a significant vital force on the body generally and gives the body strength and endurance. An adequate supply of calcium is important for building muscles, including maintenance of a strong heart muscle. Calcium has been found to activate the enzymes of the body. It is also necessary to coagulate the blood to prevent excessive bleeding, and calcium has been found to normalize the body metabolism, the process by which living organized substances are produced and maintained. The absorption of calcium into the body is aided by the presence of Vitamin D, ascorbic acid and lactose. Absorption is hindered by the presence of oxalic acid.

Result of deficiencies. Teeth and bones suffer ill effects. The bones are brittle and will break easily. The heart is weak and there is general weakness due to poor circulation. The nerves suffer and there is tenseness and irritability. Growth is poor and there is weight loss. A condition of osteoporosis or abnormal enlargement of spaces within the bone structure is apt to occur as well as osteomalacia, the condition of soft bones.

Availability. Calcium is available from cheese, skim and whole milk, cream, sea vegetation, dried figs, celery, rutabagas, dates and raisins. There are also quantities of calcium in mustard and turnip greens, as well as in kale and sesame seeds.

MINERALS—CHLORINE

Value. Chlorine, in proper quantity, keeps the joints and tendons supple. It also helps to prevent pyorrhea and excessive accumulation of fat. It will also de-toxify uneliminated matter or substances found in the body.

Result of deficiency. A deficiency of chlorine will result in excessive accumulation of waste matter, resulting in auto-intoxication or self-poisoning.

Availability. Chlorine is found in cheese, celery, cabbage, tomatoes, endive, spinach, fish, alfalfa, and sea vegetation.

MINERALS—COPPER

Value. Copper is necessary in the body for the assimilation of iron.

Result of deficiency. A deficiency in copper results in the same deficiencies which occur when iron is deficient in supply, such as anemia, pale complexion, and a general weakened condition with poor resistance to disease.

Some experiments have revealed that increasing the ingestion of copper into the body has retarded the development of cancer in animals and has decreased the liver damage caused by cancer-inducing materials. There may be reason to believe, therefore, that a deficiency in copper may contribute toward the development of cancer cells.

Availability. Copper is found in the tissues of many vegetables and animals.

MINERALS—FLUORINE

Value. Fluorine is a mineral that fights infections and is especially helpful in preventing diseases of the bone.

Result of deficiency. A deficiency in fluorine may cause pyorrhea (infection of the teeth) as well as decay of the teeth. Also, the body may more easily become infected with all types of diseases. Poor eyesight is one indication of lack of fluorine in the diet.

Availability. Fluorine is found in cow's milk, yolk of egg, and in the brains of cattle.

MINERALS—IODINE

Value. Iodine is a gland regulator, especially of the thyroid gland. Iodine protects the brain from certain body toxins and prevents simple goiter or swelling of the thyroid gland.

Result of deficiency. A deficiency of iodine may cause various gland troubles, especially the thyroid gland, and cause simple goiter or other toxic conditions.

Availability. Iodine is found in fish, dulse, various forms of sea vegetation, and in small quantities in grapes, cranberries, oranges, mushrooms, cabbage, celery, carrots, cucumbers and lettuce. Of course, should soil be deficient in iodine, there will be a lesser quantity of this mineral in the vegetables.

MINERALS—IRON

Value. Iron gives vitality to the body, building red blood cells and thus helping to carry oxygen throughout the blood system. It is regarded as an important blood salt.

Result of deficiencies. Lack of iron may cause anemia, pale face, general weakness, and lowered resistance to disease germs.

Availability. Iron is found in egg yolk, whole wheat, lean meat, sea vegetation, dried apricots, dried peaches, prunes, raisins, parsnips, cauliflower, beets, blackberries, pineapple, sweet potatoes and grapes.

MINERALS—MAGNESIUM

Value. Magnesium helps the nervous system and promotes sleep, refreshing the body generally. It is excellent for the complexion.

Result of deficiency. Nervous conditions are often due to a lack of sufficient magnesium in the diet. Another symptom is restlessness and excess acidity.

Availability. Magnesium is found in almonds, walnuts, peanuts, barley, corn, raisins, prunes, beef, fish, milk, oatmeal, raspberries, cherries, beets, dandelions, spinach, and various forms of sea vegetation.

MINERALS–MANGANESE

Value. Manganese is necessary for proper nutrition, mainly because it has the effect of activating other minerals in the body. It is known as the fertility mineral, and the lack of sufficient manganese may cause an inability to produce offspring.

Result of deficiency. A lack of sufficient manganese may cause sterility, and generally results in poor functioning of body movements.

Availability. Manganese is found in fair quantities in whole grains, rice, nuts, bananas, leafy vegetables, beets, asparagus, celery, squash, parsley, spinach, lettuce, and sea vegetation such as kelp.

MINERALS–PHOSPHORUS

Value. Phosphorus nourishes the brain and helps in the growth of bones, and is therefore of special importance for growing children. It is important for good teeth and hair. It also prevents fatigue and is therefore especially valuable for people who do considerable indoor or mental work.

Result of deficiency. A deficiency in phosphorus may cause mental fatigue, poor bone development and neurasthenia, the name for the feeling of depression resulting from exhausted nervous energy.

Availability. It is available from egg yolk, lean meat, fish, nuts, oatmeal, whole wheat, corn meal, prunes and sea vegetation.

MINERALS–POTASSIUM

Value. Potassium stimulates the liver, helps tissues to retain their elasticity, heals injured parts of the body, relieves pain, helps prevent constipation, and activates and balances chemical imbalances. It converts sugar into energy or into body starch (glycogen) to be held in storage for future energy needs.

Result of deficiency. Liver ailments result from a deficiency of potassium, and there is often constipation and pimpling of the skin. The lack of potassium may also prevent sores from healing. A lack of potassium will often cause a swelling (edema) as where there is a deficiency in potassium, sodium will enter the tissue cells and take water with it. Sometimes actual paralysis of muscles will take place due to insufficient potassium, as it is vital for muscle contractions.

Availability. Potassium is found in beans, asparagus, potatoes, raisins, spinach, dates, cabbage, carrots, lettuce, tomatoes, peaches and sea plants.

MINERALS—SILICON

Value. Silicon is reported to harden the teeth, make the hair glossy, improve the eyesight and complexion, and make the body tissues strong and supple. It is also said to help keep the fingernails and toenails strong and to keep the body in good tone.

Result of deficiency. Insufficient silicon in the body may cause baldness or gray hair. It also makes it difficult to have a good skin complexion and there may be skin irritations and rashes. Hearing may be affected and the keenness of vision formerly present may slowly disappear. The teeth may become soft and start to decay.

Availability. It is found in oats, barley, spinach, asparagus, lettuce, tomatoes, cabbage, figs and strawberries.

MINERALS—SODIUM

Value. Sodium is an alkalizer or digestive chemical. It is necessary to have sodium in the body in order to use the iron. Sodium prevents catarrh and various hardening processes.

Result of deficiency. A deficiency in sodium can well result in a deficiency in iron. In addition, indigestion may be common and the hardening processes of old age, with deposits of calcium around bone joints causing arthritis and rheumatism, is more likely to take place. Deficiency of sodium may also be a contributory cause of gallbladder and kidney stones.

Availability. Sodium is available from wheat germ, spinach, okra, beets, strawberries, lima beans, pumpkins, turnips, string beans, cucumbers, carrots and sea vegetation. It is also available in oysters and clams.

MINERALS—SULFUR

Value. Sulfur is said to purify and tone the system, promoting bile secretions, and is excellent for producing glossy hair.

Result of deficiency. The lack of sufficient sulfur tends to inhibit the functioning of the liver. As a result, impurities remain in the blood.

Availability. Sulfur is found in lean meat, fish, eggs, cauliflower, broccoli, cucumbers, corn, onion, turnips and sea vegetation.

NIACIN (NICOTINIC ACID)

Value. There is a vitamin known as Niacin, which is a synonym for nicotinic acid. The chemical formula is $C_6H_5NO_2$ and this vitamin is an important part of the Vitamin B complex. It works with the other B vitamins in converting the carbohydrates (sugars and starches) into energy, and it has been singled out as an important factor in the prevention of pellagra, the deficiency disease marked by lesions, swelling, itching and nervous disturbances. This vitamin, as well as the other B vitamins, works closely with the proteins and amino acids for good health. Usually, the recommendation for the amount of niacin is that it is required by the body approximately ten times the need of the body for thiamine (Vitamin B_1).

Results of deficiency. A deficiency of niacin leads to pellagra, a skin disease (dermatitis) affecting the skin surfaces generally exposed to light or subjected to trauma (physical contacts). There may also occur severe inflammation of mucous membranes, including swelling of the tongue (covered with ulcers, tender and painful, with thick saliva and often a rise of temperature), ulcers on the cheeks and lips, with pain and bad breath, diarrhea (loose bowels) probably with inflammation of the intestines with perhaps mucus and bloody discharges, inflammation of the rectum and anus, probably with ulcerated areas and vaginitis, and the condition of inflammation of the mucous membrane, usually accompanied by ulcerated or bleeding areas or spots.

Another sign of deficiency of niacin is a mental depression usually accompanied by suspicion and hostility. Sometimes insanity in the form of actual violence may be the result. At the outset, there may be noticeable personality changes such as fear, apprehension, confusion, and a lack of desire to carry on with customary activities. Other symptoms are insomnia, indigestion, abdominal pain, dizziness, headaches, nervousness, irritability, and loss of appetite, weight and strength.

An extreme symptom of the need for nicotinic acid could be vomiting, due to the body's difficulty in digesting food swallowed by the individual with the deficiency. Testing of the bone marrow may also show an atrophy of the marrow due to the lack of this important nutrient.

Availability. Niacin (or nicotinic acid) is perhaps most abundant in peanuts. Almost equal to the peanut source is its availability rɔrı ʳaw beef liver or from brewer's yeast. Rice polishings are high in niacin, and also such foods as wheat germ, whole barley, beef steak, lobster, haddock, stewed chicken, fresh soybeans, whole bran, whole buckwheat, buttermilk, whole milk, collard greens, kale, turnip greens, potatoes, tomatoes, green peas, eggs, and mushrooms. There is a difference between niacin and niacinamide. The former causes the skin to flush and prickle and the blood vessels to dilate. This is not considered dangerous, but the use of niacinamide (a slightly different substance with substantially the same effect) as a vitamin preparation does not produce these effects. It may be safer to use the natural food products named above when they are available.

OXALIC ACID

Value. Recent research indicates that oxalic acid markedly reduces the blood coagulation time, making it valuable in treating conditions where there is uncontrolled bleeding or hemorrhages. Often individuals will avoid many fine fruits and vegetables because there is some oxalic acid in them and they may have passed some calcium-oxalate stones. However, it has been found that oxalate stones are formed even when no oxalic acid whatsoever is in the diet. Apparently stones will form from a deficiency in Vitamin A, and there are undoubtedly other factors about body chemistry in regard to stone formation that are still unknown. A shortage of Vitamin B_6 has also been associated with calcium-oxalate stone formation. It has been suggested that no healthful food should be avoided but emphasis placed on complete protein and mineral balances, and to avoid deficiencies of any of the important nutrients.

Results of deficiency. Little is known about the results of deficiency of oxalic acid. Rather, in view of the history of stone formation attributed to this acid, the emphasis seems to be to learn how to avoid an excessive amount. Our knowledge of the chemistry of nutrition is really not precise enough to tell us at this time whether oxalic acid is a friend or a foe.

Availability. Oxalic acid is found in almost all fruits and vegetables, and especially in spinach. This is not to say that spinach should be avoided, as there is doubt as to whether or not the presence of oxalic acid has any major effect upon nutrition in normal circumstances. Where an individual has not been obtaining the desired balance of nutrients, then, of course, anything can happen. The more common sources are cranberries, chard, rhubarb, gooseberries, spinach, and beet leaves. Authorities advise that when these foods are eaten, the large amounts of oxalic acid will probably be neutralized by partaking of such foods as eggs, beans and milk.

PARA-AMINO-BENZOIC ACID (PABA)

Value. This is another B vitamin. Its chemical formula is $C_7H_7NO_2$ and it is slightly soluble in water, stable in dilute acid and alkali, and easily oxidized. It is one of the components of folic acid and helps to maintain the natural color of the hair, as well as helping to maintain the reproductive glands and organs. A number of authorities recommend as much as 200 mg. of this vitamin daily. PABA has been recognized as having an inhibitory influence upon the growth of the minute organisms, probably protozoa, found in typhus fever, Rocky Mountain spotted fever and trench fever, a condition known as Rickettsia. It is also known to inhibit the growth of other bacteria and exerts an inhibitive influence upon the thyroid hormone synthesis. As the thyroid produces only one hormone, thyroxine, which is rich in iodine and which accelerates the metabolism of all cells and tissues, it is important for the thyroid to function properly.

Some time ago, a physician in Bucharest, Roumania, Dr. Anna Aslan, made the statement that para-amino-benzoic acid, which she labeled as H_3, would revitalize the body, producing a youthful resurgence when taken over a period of time. Her reports and the reports of other physicians indicated that in many cases of arthritis PABA has been of material assistance, and has also strengthened muscles, relieved severe body pains, stopped twitching muscles, and even improved the memory. Best of all, one report indicated the restoration of an optimistic outlook and a feeling of well-being.

Another value for PABA is its reported effective use as a sunburn preventative when applied externally to the skin prior to exposure or ingesting it daily to the extent of 1,000 milligrams. It is also valuable in removing the pain of sunburn or other burns to the body. There are indications that when used as a skin cream it may delay the skin changes usually accompanying the aging process.

Results of deficiency. A deficiency may result in loss of hair or failure of hair to grow. There may also exist an inability to produce offspring. The lack of or insufficient PABA may prevent normal functioning of the various glands and organs of the body, and the presence of this vitamin controls the growth of undesirable bacteria or protozoa found in typhus fever, Rocky Mountain spotted fever, and trench fever. A lack of PABA may also be a contributory factor in producing hyperthyroidism, as its presence controls the action of the thyroid gland.

Availability. It is readily available from the foods that ordinarily have the B-complex vitamins, and such foods as rice polish, rice bran and wheat germ are especially valuable for this vitamin. It is also found in yeast, liver and kidneys.

PROTEINS AND ESSENTIAL AMINO ACIDS

Proteins comprise amino acids, of which there are approximately twenty-two in number. Some of the amino acids can be manufactured by the body itself, but certain amino acids must be present in the diet. These are called essential amino acids, as follows:

1. Histidine	6. Phenylalanine
2. Isoleucine	7. Tryptophan
3. Leucine	8. Valine
4. Lysine	9. Threonine
5. Methionine	

Some foods may contain some of these essential amino acids but others may be lacking. Thus it is often necessary to eat foods in combination with each other so that the body will obtain the necessary nourishment.

While the accepted standard minimum requirement of 25 to 40 grams of protein is given, it must be noted that this applies to the adult who is in normal good health and only if the protein is of excellent quality. In addition, there must be no drain on the protein supply for calories needed by the body and therefore there must be an adequate bodily intake of carbohydrate and fat.

Individuals who undertake fad or crash diets in efforts to quickly

DAILY PROTEIN NEEDS OF INDIVIDUALS

Body size	Minimum Requirement	Recommended Allowance	Comment
	(in grams)	(in grams)	
Male Adult Average size	25-40	75	
Woman Adult Average size	25-40	60	20 grams additional during pregnancy and 40 grams if a nursing mother.
Infant		1 to 1½ per lb.	
Child 6-9 53 lbs.		52	
Teen-ager girl or boy		75-100	

reduce excessive weight will often curtail drastically the intake of protein, whereas such individuals need above-normal quantities of protein in order to cope with the stress and strain of drastic dieting.

Likewise, elderly people must be warned not to curtail their protein intake, as rebuilding and repair of tissue continues throughout life.

PROTEIN AND THE DIGESTIVE PROCESS

When food enters the stomach, it meets with the gastric (stomach) juices, such as hydrochloric acid, and pepsin, an enzyme. These juices transform molecules of protein into smaller molecules, which in turn are acted upon by juices from the pancreas and the intestinal wall, the enzymes trypsin and erepsin, to again transform the smaller molecules into amino acids.

The amino acids enter into the blood circulation and are then carried to the liver and other tissues of the body, and serve the purpose of repairing and replacing cells of the body. Because there is a continuous wear and tear of body cells, protein is needed by the body to serve the purpose of maintaining the individual in good health.

For each gram of protein food, there are approximately four calories of heat or energy. If the body does not obtain enough calories from fat or carbohydrate items of diet, the body will use the calories found in protein to provide the bodily needs for heat and energy. When this happens, unless there are ample protein foods in the system, the protein in the body will be used to furnish heat and energy (as calories) instead of being used to build or replace body tissue. The body does not store protein. The liver will automatically take excess protein and remove the nitrogen from it. The remaining molecule is then used either as a source of energy or is stored as fat. Thus, contrary to common belief, excessive protein can result in excessive fat build-ups even when fat as a food is carefully avoided.

Proteins (also referred to as proteids) are divided into animal and vegetable categories, with no important difference between the two classes. They all contain carbon, hydrogen, nitrogen and oxygen, and are subdivided into (1) albumins, (2) globulins, (3) albuminates or derived albumins, (4) proteoses, (5) peptones, and (6) coagulated proteids. Unless one is a chemist or professional nutritionist, it is not really necessary to an understanding of proteins to study such details as their precipitation, coagulation, saturation and solubility points and other technical details.

The average person should, however, understand the need for an adequate protein consumption, the minimum daily requirements, the conditions for which increased protein intake is required, and the various common sources of protein. We shall try to cover these matters briefly and accurately.

The National Research Council reports that each individual needs .9 grams of protein for each 2.2 pounds of body weight. For practical purposes, and to make it easier to estimate the amount of protein a person should consume daily, the rule might be stated simply as one gram of protein for each two pounds of body weight. For example, a person weighing 150 pounds would need approximately 75 grams of protein daily.

Growing children, pregnant women, nursing mothers, and persons in need of special care due to illness such as anemia may need special diets with increased amounts of protein. The needs vary greatly, depending upon circumstances. The man of average weight and height may get along nicely with 75 grams of protein daily, and the average woman of a weight of approximately 125 pounds may have an adequate supply of protein by taking 60 grams daily. The pregnant woman, during the second half of her pregnancy, needs to provide her infant with nutrients from her blood, so she should take an extra supply of protein, for a total of perhaps 85 grams daily. Likewise, growing boys and girls of the ages from 13 to 20 years should partake of protein to the extent of from 75 to 100 grams daily.

The most common sources of protein are dried soybeans, pignolia nuts, pumpkin and squash seed, wheat germ, peanuts, dulse, dried lentils, dried mung beans, dried peas, sunflower seeds, almonds, sesame seeds, wild rice, dried hot red pepper, and many other foods as listed in this encyclopedia. Practically all foods have some protein value but the foods listed have the highest quantity of protein of comparable quality.

VITAMINS AND MINERALS

The official government position with regard to the difference between natural and synthetic vitamins has been explained in one of the Yearbooks of the United States Department of Agriculture. A government biochemist, George M. Briggs, explained that natural foods have "several important nutrients and substances whose identity we still do not know. We call them unidentified factors."

In studies of the growth and reproduction of animals, it has been found that the superior growth resulting from the use of natural food products "cannot be duplicated with pure protein or amino acids." The isolation of unidentified factors requires long periods of expensive laboratory studies. Briggs stated that "the grass juice factor is a good example of how long studies on unidentified factors often take. It takes particularly devoted scientists to stick to a problem, for example, that goes on for twenty years without an answer."

It has taken many years to isolate the various categories of B vitamins, and scientists are still recognizing and isolating additional B vitamins. It is obviously more desirable to eat some brewer's yeast or other natural substance which contains all of the B vitamins, both known and unknown, rather than to purchase a few isolated vitamins that have been presently identified.

In some instances, in the course of processing of foods, a manufacturer will remove vitamins during the process of manufacturing and will "enrich" the resultant product by adding one, two, or three vitamins. Many of the vitamins that are used in the enrichment process have been obtained from the synthesizing of coal or wood-tar derivitives, and for that reason may actually be toxic. In addition, the "enrichment" of a product by the addition of fewer than the original number of vitamins may easily produce a deficiency, as in many cases vitamins must be ingested into the body in proper proportions. It is, therefore, wiser and safer to eat natural foods and to avoid the risks of depending upon obtaining an adequate supply of vitamins from the pill bottles or from the so-called "enriched" foods.

Minerals, too, are available in natural foods, and whenever possible the natural minerals should be absorbed into the system rather than minerals bottled specially by man. It has been found that by partaking of a diet of completely natural foods we can avoid mineral deficiencies that result when minerals are taken in tablet or capsule form. It has been found that some of the minerals react with other foods in such a way as to be lost because they become insoluble or become saponified, which is a form of chemical decomposition. Some minerals, unfortunately, are distributed only over a portion of the earth's surface. Consequently, they can be found only in foods grown in the places where these minerals are part of the soil.

Where there is any lack of natural foods containing the natural minerals and vitamins, it is then important that the individual provide his body with these nutrients, preferably from naturally derived sources. But it should be remembered that whenever possible, the vitamins and minerals as contained in the natural foods are best for the body.

Throughout this encyclopedia, the nutritive values of all natural foods such as fruits, vegetables, nuts and seeds are fully explained. With the aid of the index, one can find which natural foods will provide the vitamins or minerals needed. The index is especially valuable when one wishes to ascertain just which foods contain some particular vitamin or mineral.

VITAMIN A

Value. This vitamin has a special relationship to the "lining cells" of the body, including the skin, eyes, urinary tract, bones, teeth, and the gastrointestinal tract (pertaining to the stomach and intestines). It is also known as an anti-infection vitamin, helping the body to fight off disease. This vitamin is an essential constituent of the pigments which the retina of the eye uses to register visual stimuli.

Results of deficiency. A lack of Vitamin A affects the skin, the digestive system, respiratory tract, genito-urinary system, special senses, and the glandular system of the body. The skin will probably become rough and dry. Also bones are affected, so that growing children will have problems with bone formation, bone repair and faulty tooth formation. Insufficient Vitamin A is likely to decrease the amount of acid required by the stomach to digest food, and diarrhea may be an obvious symptom.

There may also be an inability to gain weight, and in fact there is likely to be a decrease in weight. The hair may start to fall out and become gray, and there may be a disposition toward abscesses of the scalp. Small pus formations (pustules) may form on the scalp and on other parts of the skin. The forearms and the thighs will be especially noticeable for the roughness and scaliness.

Lack of this vitamin will make a person inclined toward cystitis (inflammation of the bladder, marked by painful passage of urine), pyelitis (inflammation of the pelvis of the kidney), urethritis (inflammation of the urethra), and there is likely to develop stones in the kidney and bladder. Pus cells will often form and be excreted in the urine. The condition known as senile vaginitis may occur, where raw spots in the vagina develop, and these spots may adhere to opposite surfaces, blocking the vaginal canal. A deficiency in this vitamin may also cause muscular degeneration (atrophy of muscular tissue, including the muscular tissue of the heart), as well as degeneration of the spinal cord, often accompanied by disseminated sclerosis, the form of disease where there are many hardened patches dispersed throughout the brain and spinal cord.

The eyes are especially vulnerable to a Vitamin A deficiency. The malnutrition of the eyes and appurtenant tissues makes it especially difficult to see well under trying conditions, especially at night. There is difficulty in tolerating bright lights and often there is an itching, burning, and dryness of the eyes, perhaps accompanied by dancing specks and flashes. The impaired vision is usually accompanied by eyestrain, often with the presence of sticky secretions and granulations in the eyes. Often there is an inflammation of the delicate membrane which lines the lids and covers the eyeball, the condition termed conjunctivitis.

The lack of this vitamin often leads to infection of the middle ear, which may affect a person's hearing. There may also be a degeneration of the mucous membrane of the nose, making it easier for bacteria to take hold, with resultant infections. The mouth and throat is similarly liable to infection when Vitamin A is in short supply. One of the signs of shortage of Vitamin A is a scarcity of saliva in the mouth. The teeth will have a tendency to decay more easily and the tooth enamel will become defective.

A deficiency of Vitamin A affects the respiratory system by such signs as a dry cough, hoarseness of the voice, and a disposition to colds and infection of the sinus area. In addition, there is likely to be bronchitis and pneumonia.

There is often a lack of vitality when this vitamin deficiency exists, as well as an inferior appetite and intestinal disturbances. Nursing mothers having this vitamin deficiency will produce insufficient milk for their children.

Other studies indicate that a lack of Vitamin A in the diet of the male will make him sterile and unable to reproduce due to atrophy of the testes. Also, a cleft palate and harelip may be due to a Vitamin A deficiency.

Availability. This vitamin is available from many fruits, vegetables; nuts and seeds, as well as in cod and halibut-liver oil, chicken and calf liver, egg yolk, cheese, whole milk and butter. For vegetarians or persons who prefer obtaining Vitamin A from fruits and vegetables, carrot juice is high in this vitamin, as well as parsley, spinach, beet greens, mustard greens, kale, lamb's quarters, endive, oxalis (stemless herb), dandelion greens, turnip greens, broccoli, apricots, lettuce, cabbage, watercress, peaches, peas, beans, papayas, sweet potatoes, dried prunes, asparagus, sweet corn, oranges, cantaloupes, pecans, and many other foods. Refer to the various food listings for the exact quantity of this vitamin in each food.

VITAMIN B₁

Value. Vitamin B₁ is also known as thiamin or thiamine. However, there are several vitamins in the B complex, and they are all interdependent and should all be taken at the same time. A failure to have all of the B complex vitamins may lower the body's resistance to disease. Thiamine is especially valuable as an aid in the metabolism of carbohydrates. Unless carbohydrates can be converted into energy, the individual will lack energy, drive and sparkle. This vitamin is considered essential for reproductive powers and for proper nerve function.

Results of deficiency. An insufficient supply of thiamine can result in a variety of symptoms related to the functioning of the nervous system, such as irritability, insomnia, loss of appetite and constipation. At times the arms and legs may feel numb due to the unhealthy nerves. The lack of sufficient thiamine may cause beriberi, the disease marked by extreme weakness, loss of appetite and weight, digestive disturbance, painful neuritis, and even paralysis. The heart action is likely to become abnormal and mental depression is a common symptom. The individual becomes short of breath with but very little exertion. An insufficient supply of this vitamin also prevents the formation of hydrochloric acid in the stomach, which is needed for digestion of food. Thiamine is a part of the enzyme system that breaks down pyruvic and lactic acids, releasing energy.

Another symptom of this deficiency is a constant craving for sweets. This is due to the failure of the body to obtain energy from sugars, starches and carbohydrates in the digestive system, as thiamine is needed for the conversion of these foods into energy. Consequently, the body is always hungry and the individual constantly craves sweets or other rich foods in an effort to meet the hunger needs. Unfortunately, the erroneous thinking among many people is that as thiamine removes the loss of appetite (one of the symptoms of thiamine deficiency), it should be avoided. However, by avoiding thiamine the body lacks energy, and as a result there is an increase in desire for food, especially sweets, in an effort to satisfy the body requirements for energy.

One of the first signs of Vitamin B$_1$ deficiency is a slow pulse, perhaps not more than 40 to 50 beats a minute. The blood pressure also falls below normal but occasionally the heart will increase it's speed, apparently due to irritation of the heart muscle by accumulations of pyruvic acid. A Vitamin B$_1$ deficiency may also result in the development of an enlarged heart, especially where an individual is actively working at hard labor or is engaged in strenuous athletics. When the heart slows down, the digestive tract becomes sluggish and food is incompletely digested, resulting in constipation. The food waste stays too long in the intestinal tract, gas forms, and the intestinal tract becomes dry and the contents harden.

As this vitamin is water-soluble, only a small amount is stored in the body and therefore it should be replenished daily. A minimum quantity to take daily is from 1.0 to 1.4 milligrams, but for a margin of safety one should aim for a minimum of from three to four milligrams daily. As it is water-soluble, the vitamin is lost when the food containing it is soaked or cooked in water and the water then discarded.

Ordinary cooking does not destroy this vitamin but, as indicated, it dissolves into the water in which it is being cooked. It does not dissolve in the presence of oils and fats. Tests indicate that the soda usually added to vegetables to keep them fresh and green destroys this vitamin.

Another indication of a deficiency in this vitamin is a feeling of nausea, sometimes accompanied by vomiting, loss of appetite and headaches. There may also be general weakness, muscle pains and cramps, atrophy of muscles, and a warm, pink, flushed skin. A lack of muscular coordination may be noticeable, the condition known as ataxia. Some areas of the skin may be excessively sensitive and the various reflexes may be diminished. In addition, there may be a swelling or edema of the arms and legs, with swelling of several nerves (polyneuritis) and a sensation of burning of feet. The pupils of the eyes may dilate and there may be ear noises and impairment of the vocal cords that may cause hoarseness or loss of voice entirely. Severe deficiency may cause fainting and the customary symptoms of anemia may appear. In addition, there may be pulmonary congestion with difficult breathing and the skin turning blue. The memory may become defective and in extreme cases the individual may suffer extreme nervous agitation and fearful hallucinations, as in the case of severe alcoholic addiction.

Availability. The richest source of Vitamin B_1 is wheat germ. There are also ample quantities in brewer's yeast, whole raw barley, peanut flour, soybean flour, whole-wheat flour, human milk, whole buckwheat, livers and hearts of beef, green raw peas and many other foods, such as whole wheat bread, egg yolks, rye bread, black walnuts, roasted peanuts, Brazil nuts, pecans and hazel nuts.

VITAMIN B₂

Value. Vitamin B_2, also known as Vitamin G, was discovered in 1932 and given its name and identity in 1937. It's chemical formula is $C_{17}H_{20}N_4O_6$. It is also known as riboflavin. It is an important factor in growth and development of the body and promotes a healthy condition of the skin. It is especially valuable in combination with Vitamin A for prevention and correction of cataracts and for health of the skin, hair and eyes. This vitamin is also important to the body in assimilating iron and proteins. Being water-soluble, it is not easily stored in the body. It is affected by light but not by air or heat.

An important chemical function of this vitamin is to break down starches and sugars into energy, a function similar to that of Vitamin B_1. This enables the body to better resist infectious disease and is necessary for good health and vitality. An ample supply of this vitamin will help produce healthier offspring and delay the bodily changes that often accompany increasing years of life. It is said that the centenarians of Bulgaria have a diet rich in Vitamin B_2.

Results of deficiency. A lack of Vitamin B_2 may cause inflammation of the membrane of the eye and eyelids (conjunctivitis), lips that become sore and red and later cracked and peeled, especially at the mouth corners. Often, the first sign of deficiency is dimness of vision at a distance or in poor light. The cornea (the white, glasslike area of the eyeball) may become bloodshot and inflamed if the deficiency is allowed to continue. The theory is that this vitamin carries oxygen, and when no oxygen arrives the body forms new blood vessels to bring oxygen to the parts lacking it. An absence of riboflavin produced cataracts in experimentations.

Other indications of a need for this vitamin are lack of appetite, painful cramps in abdomen and stomach, inability to gain weight, loss of weight, reddening, scaliness and roughness of the skin. There is often difficulty in walking, with muscular weakness and stiffness. Crusts may form on the skin of the face, especially around the nose and on the scalp. The scalp condition is commonly known as dandruff, the scales falling from the scalp when they accumulate in large amounts. As there may be a disposition to infection of the middle ear, there may be a deterioration in hearing as an indication of deficiency of this vitamin. In addition, the skin of the ears may develop a greasy skin with red scales. Also, the skin may crack at the fingernails.

Another indication of a deficiency in Vitamin B_2 may be a dark red or purplish tongue, also somewhat swollen and granulated. In addition, the individual may have an anemic or pale and thin appearance, and the reproductive functions will probably be poor due to glandular disequilibrium and generally poor assimilation of other food taken into the digestive system.

This vitamin is little affected by heat, so cooking operations do not destroy it. It is soluble in water but is unstable in alkaline solutions and may decompose in a strong alkaline environment. In experiments with animals, it was found that doses one thousand times normal produced no toxic effects. This vitamin is sensitive to light and is damaged when exposed to strong light. On the other hand, persons lacking this vitamin become sensitive to strong lights and find it difficult to tolerate such lighting.

Availability. A minimum of from four to five milligrams each day of this vitamin should be sought. Apparently, individuals need about twenty-five or fifty percent more of Vitamin B_2 than of Vitamin B_1. Glandular meats, such as that of the heart, liver or kidney, are high in this vitamin, with calf liver leading the list. For the vegetarians, sizeable quantities of this vitamin are available from broccoli, both leaf and flower, raw collards, and from leafy green vegetables generally. The outer green leaves of lettuce and cabbage contain at least five times as much of the vitamin as the inside leaves.

Other sources of Vitamin B_2 are the tops of turnips, beets and dandelions. In addition, wheat germ provides this vitamin as well as peanuts, blueberries, dried prunes, cheese, eggs, apples, watercress, carrots, coconuts, grapefruit and lemons. This vitamin is also available from whole milk, whole wheat bread, fish, and poultry. While beef generally contains this vitamin, the glandular parts of beef meat, as previously indicated, are more richly supplied with riboflavin.

VITAMIN B_6

Value. Another important factor in the prevention of tooth decay is Vitamin B_6. This vitamin, also known as pyridoxine, has a soothing or sedative effect on the nerves and so it is of great value to people who wish to avoid nervousness. This vitamin is of great value in maintaining the tone of the muscles, and of course the heart is a muscle and is immediately affected by a deficiency in this vitamin. It is also of value in maintaining a normal blood count with an ample supply of hemoglobin, the coloring substance of the red blood corpuscles.

In experiments with animals, it has been learned that Vitamin B_6 is important for proper functioning of the pancreas. If the pancreas sustains damage so that it cannot produce insulin, the hormone necessary for conversion of sugar (glucose) into energy, diabetes may be the result.

Results of deficiency. A deficiency in pyridoxine may result in an excessively oily skin, dizziness, tension, insomnia, fatigue, irritability, nervousness, stiffness of the legs, palsy or trembling of limbs, known as Parkinson's disease, swollen, red and sore skin, drooping shoulders and backs, a shuffling walk instead of normal walking and, in the case of pregnant women, dizziness, morning sickness and nausea. Travelers are more apt to suffer from car, train, sea and plane sickness when this vitamin is in short supply. The tongue and the area under the tongue may develop ulcers and lesions may develop in the throat and around the mouth. Experiments indicate that there is apt to be retarded growth, depressed appetite and poor utilization of food that is ingested. The final result of the deficiency is death, preceded by convulsions. The sedative effect of this vitamin upon the nerves has prompted its use in epilepsy cases and there have been some favorable responses in cases of muscular dystrophy.

While in many cases a deficiency of this vitamin will cause tension and nervousness, there have been reports that deficiency may also cause a mental depression with extreme weakness of muscles and with some of the other symptoms previously mentioned, such as dizziness and nausea.

Some investigators have reported that a deficiency of this vitamin may cause a rash or dermatitis in the vagina, with swelling, itching, bleeding and inflammation. Where a deficiency causes skin diseases and deterioration of the mucous membrane linings within the internal parts of the body, it is safe to assume that diarrhea, inflammation of the intestines and especially of the colon (colitis) may be due in part at least to a deficiency in Vitamin B_6.

It should be noted, incidentally, that the body needs magnesium in order to utilize Vitamin B_6, and although an individual's diet may be sufficient for the vitamin, the lack of magnesium may render the taking of the vitamin useless.

Among other symptoms of Vitamin B_6 deficiency are vomiting, gas in stomach and intestines, eczema, respiratory infections and anemia. There is danger that individuals suffering from anemia may be given large doses of iron without consideration for the need of Vitamin B_6 to maintain the normal blood count. Excessive iron supplies may damage the tissues and unless accompanied by adequate amounts of Vitamin B_6 death may result.

The absence of this vitamin may also cause severe atherosclerosis, with the arteries in the heart, pancreas, kidneys, abdomen, limbs, muscles, and all tissues becoming clogged with fatty deposits. When the pancreas cannot function well, its ability to supply insulin for the control of carbohydrates is damaged and a lack of insulin is the immediate cause of diabetes mellitus.

The loss of hair may also be the result of deficiency of this vitamin. Another reported condition resulting from this deficiency is hemorrhoids, usually corrected rather quickly when this vitamin is restored to the diet. For some reason, pregnant women are often deficient in the supply of this vitamin and often suffer from bleeding in the area of the anus.

Availability. Vitamin B_6 is available from the consumption of liver, kidney, heart, corn oil, brewer's yeast, honey, egg yolk, cabbage, whole grain cereals, whole grain breads and fish.

VITAMIN B_{12}

Value. This vitamin is essential for the blood-forming organs of the bone marrow if they are to function properly. Also, the nervous system depends upon this vitamin for nutrition. One of the ingredients of this vitamin is cobalt, and it appears from the study of scientific materials that Vitamin B_{12} is now being referred to as cobalamin, because of the importance of cobalt in the diet. Likewise, zinc is associated with this vitamin, the studies indicating that the vitamin cannot be synthesized without the help of zinc. Vitamin B_{12} is also needed to help form hemoglobin, as good red blood should score 100 on the hemoglobin scale. Thus this vitamin is important for the prevention of anemia. It also combines with folic acid to help produce the vital red blood cells. Actually, it has been stated that less than one millionth of a gram of cobalamin is needed daily to meet the human body requirements.

Results of deficiency. The lack of cobalamin may cause pernicious anemia, due to the inability of the bone marrow to form blood when this vitamin is absent. A symptom of lack of cobalamin is a shuffling gait. Another indication is a loss of sense of position of the feet. In severe cases, where there has been a degeneration of the spinal cord, there may be nerve and brain damage and even complete paralysis.

Another result of this deficiency is general malnutrition, marked by an insufficient production of sex hormones with the resultant lack of development or shriveling of the breasts, ovaries and other sex organs. The sexual characteristics of the individual will also suffer, the female becoming less feminine and the male less manly. Among the women there will probably be irregular menstruation, a decrease in the flow or even a complete cessation, although normal menstruation may take place when the missing vitamin is supplied. Women suffering from a foul-smelling vaginal discharge may possibly have brought about the condition by failing to obtain cobalimin in their diets.

Availability. This vitamin is found mainly in liver, kidney, muscle meats, oysters, milk, eggs, cheese and salt-water fish. Of the vegetable foods, yeast, wheat germ and soybeans have cobalimin content, but only small traces of it. Vegetarians are therefore at a distinct disadvantage so far as utilizing this vitamin is concerned unless they obtain some cobalimin before it is too late.

VITAMIN C

Value. Vitamin C (ascorbic acid) is important for the supporting tissues of the body such as the cartilage, bone, teeth and connective tissues. In tests made of both natural Vitamin C as occurring in various foods and of synthetic ascorbic acid produced in laboratories by the combination of chemicals, it was found that animals having Vitamin C deficiencies were unaffected when treated with the synthetic product but that the group of animals treated with the naturally derived Vitamin C were promptly cured. This vitamin is highly sensitive to heat and its valuable properties may be destroyed by heat, air, alkali or enzymes. Acid tends to preserve and protect this vitamin, while the presence of copper accelerates its destruction. It is important in the metabolism of some of the amino acids (proteins) and its greatest concentration is in most of the active tissues of the body. The average adult should obtain from 70 to 75 mg. of this vitamin each day, and the average child should have between 30 and 100 mg. depending upon the age and physical activity of the child. The older the child and the more active, the more Vitamin C he or she should have to support the body tissues.

An important value of Vitamin C is to help in the formation of collagen, a protective substance constituting about 40 percent of the body's protein, which holds our cells in a healthy and natural formation of firmly walled tissue. This helps the tissue to resist penetration by any invading infections.

Some authorities believe that massive doses of Vitamin C may be taken safely to combat any infectious body condition. A massive does would be 1000 mg. or more at a time. This would be repeated at hourly intervals until the symptoms of the disease disappear.

Result of deficiency: One of the signs of a deficiency of Vitamin C is bleeding gums. Also, a tendency to bruise easily is another sign, with profuse bleeding from minor cuts on the skin another sign. The bones will develop poorly, the cartilages will be weak, muscles will degenerate and become weak, anemia will probably appear, and there will be considerable susceptibility to all kinds of infections, colds, etc. The well-known disease named scurvy, marked by loss of energy, pain in the legs, limbs and joints, and loosening of teeth, results from insufficient Vitamin C. The British sailors found they could avoid these symptoms at sea by taking limes with them on their ships. This is how the term "Limey" first became applied to British sailors.

Availability. In the order of highest intensity, Vitamin C is available from Acerola juice, Acerola cherries, red pepper, common guava, hot green pepper, sweet red pepper and black currant. It is also available in fairly large quantities from kale leaves, parsley, collard leaves, orange peel (the part of the orange usually discarded), turnip greens, mustard spinach, sweet green pepepr, dock (sorrel), broccoli, Brussels sprouts, raw horse-radish, watercress, cauliflower and many other fruits, vegetables, nuts and seeds. Vitamin C is also found in the citrus fruits such as oranges, lemons and grapefruits. Also, tomatoes contain some Vitamin C.

VITAMIN D

Value. This vitamin promotes normal bone and tooth development and regulates the absorption and fixation of calcium and phosphorus. It is soluble in fat and is not materially affected by heat or oxidation. It is stored in the liver and synthesized in the skin by activity of ultraviolet light. Vitamin D apparently controls the blood content of calcium and phosphorus, and thus is directly related to the structure of the bones and teeth. This vitamin is necessary not only during the early years, but the absence of the vitamin causes morbid softening of the bone in adults. It is therefore of great importance for pregnant women, who are in need of greater than usual supplies of the vitamin so that they will not lose the calcium needed for the tissues and the teeth. Because of the healthy effect upon the skin, Vitamin D is essential to prevent such skin diseases as acne and psoriasis. Studies indicate that the vitamin is a factor in tissue cell respiration and that it is essential to maintain a normal basal metabolism. Authorities differ as to the amount to be ingested or absorbed daily, but studies indicate that a quantity of from 2,500 to 5,000 International Units daily would be satisfactory.

Results of deficiency. The disease of metabolism known as rickets has been often said to be the result of Vitamin D deficiency.

Symptoms are restlessness and slight fever at night (100° to 102°), free perspiration about the head, soreness of muscles generally, tenderness in numerous places, a white pallor, slight diarrhea, enlargement of liver and spleen, eruption of badly formed teeth, constipation, lordosis (curvature of spine forward) and scoliosis (spine curvature toward left and right sides).

Availability. Vitamin D is available from sunshine, which is why it is so often referred to as the "sunshine vitamin." It is also obtainable through ultra-violet radiation as well as from fish oils such as cod and halibut. Smaller amounts are also present in eggs, herring, sardines, tuna and salmon. It is also present in Vitamin D-fortified milk.

VITAMIN E

Value. Vitamin E is needed to maintain normal red blood cells especially for babies, premature and full term. Abnormalities in the blood of babies were found to exist mainly because cow's milk rather than human milk was fed to them. Tests revealed that Vitamin E in human milk was two to four times greater than in cow's milk. This vitamin is also considered vital for proper functioning of the reproductive organs, testing indicating that the absence of this vitamin produced sterility in males.

An important function of this vitamin is its ability to act on excess fat so that it will be more readily oxidized and converted into energy. This may explain why bread and butter go so well together. The Vitamin E in the bread is present to help convert the butter-fat into energy.

Some reports indicate that Vitamin E will protect the body generally from infection and that this protection will extend even to viruses. The theory presented is that the virus, on attacking body cells, interferes with the normal metabolism that takes place wherein food and oxygen is transported to body tissues. Vitamin E apparently has an inherent ability to supply oxygen to the cells, thus assisting in the metabolism, nourishing the cells and thereby enabling them to better fight off the attacking virus.

Other reports indicate that Vitamin E may be of value in cases of diabetes because of the tissue-building power of this vitamin. Some writers also report that Vitamin E seems to lower the blood pressure, correct heart disorders, and normalize most body processes and glandular functions, including the pancreas.

Results of deficiency. A deficiency in this vitamin may make it difficult for infants to survive babyhood. In addition, the lack of sufficient vitamins of this type may prevent males from having the ability to produce offspring.

One of the symptoms of a deficiency in Vitamin E is a slow deterioration of the nervous system, resulting in nervousness, irritability, headaches and fatigue. For youngsters, there will be a slow growth and development of the body with probably defective development of male reproductive cells.

Among women, a deficiency in Vitamin E may result in lack of fertility and a tendency to habitual abortion or miscarriage when pregnancy does occur. There may also be an absence of menstruation, young women may be late in maturing, and ovulation (discharge of ovum from the ovary) may be infrequent instead of the usual thirteen times a year.

Availability. This vitamin is found in various plant oils such as corn oil, cottonseed oil and wheat germ oils. It is also found in whole grain cereals as well as in lettuce, brown rice, barley, rye, wheat germ, rice germ, various green leaves of vegetables, nuts and legumes, such as beans, lentils and peas, and egg yolk.

VITAMIN F

Value. This vitamin promotes growth and is known as the unsaturated fatty acids. This fatty acid, rather than the saturated fatty acid, is of value to the body as offering the most concentrated form of energy. Unsaturated fatty acids combine with phosphorus to form part of every cell and are particularly concentrated in nerve and brain tissues. A thin padding of fat lies directly under the skin, serves as cushioning for the nerves and muscles, and when there are sudden changes of temperature the layer of fat protects the body from the effect of such sudden changes. These acids are also valuable in preventing high cholesterol buildups in the arteries.

Results of deficiency. Some of the symptoms of lack of unsaturated fatty acids include emaciation, severe skin rashes, kidney disorders, difficulty in healing of even small wounds, interference with the ability to reproduce, and shortening of the life span. Vegetarians, for example, who scrupulously avoid all fatty foods, become thin and emaciated, and practically all glands and organs of the body suffer from such extremism.

Availability. Good sources of unsaturated fatty acids include peanut oil, olive oil, all vegetable oils, butter, cream, egg yolk, nuts, avocado, fish-liver oil, fish fat and animal fat.

VITAMIN H (BIOTIN)

Value. This vitamin is a factor in the B group of vitamins and is also called biotin. It is believed to be a powerful cellular stimulant. Together with a substance found in the white of eggs, avertin, the combination of the stimulant, biotin, with the depressant, avertin, serves as a cellular balance to obtain a chemical equilibrium. A minimum of 0.1 mg. per day has been recommended.

Result of deficiency. An absence of this factor or the absence of avertin usually causes disease, as the two factors need to be balanced in the body. A deficiency in biotin may cause pathologic changes in the skin and tongue, loss of appetite, nausea, low grade anemia, with lassitude, intense depression, sleeplessness and muscle pain. Animals studied with this deficiency grew poorly, developed a general dermatitis, muscular incoordination, and hair loss.

Availability. Biotin is widely distributed in foods known to be good sources of the other B complex vitamins. Some biotin-rich foods are egg yolk, liver and yeast.

VITAMIN K

Value. This vitamin is needed in the blood for establishment of a minimum clotting time to prevent hemorrhages in the event of a cut or wound. Usually, for most people, one-half milligram per day of this vitamin is sufficient. It is customary to give this vitamin to pregnant women to add to the usually sparse supply of the vitamin in the newborn child. In surgical operations, the presence of Vitamin K in adequate amounts helps the healing processes where blood vessels have been cut in tissues.

Results of deficiency. A deficiency in this vitamin could cause excessive loss of blood in the event of a cut or other wound resulting in bleeding. In addition, a shortage of this vitamin may contribute toward the bile pigment, bilirubin, to be diffused into the blood. Symptoms of this condition, jaundice, are dark urine, light feces, fatigue, loss of appetite, general itching and slow heart action. A contributory factor in jaundice cases is the ingestion of excessive fat in the diet.

Availability. Leafy vegetables are the most common source of this vitamin. It is also manufactured in the intestines by certain bacteria. It is also found in fats, fishmeal, oats, wheat, rye and alfalfa.

VITAMIN P

Value. This vitamin, also known as citron, is antiscorbutic, helping to prevent scurvy, the disease resulting from lack of fresh fruits and vegetables. It is helpful in strengthening the walls of the capillaries, thus preventing water from seeping through into the tissues as in cases of dropsy, where watery fluid enters into tissues or cavities of the body. It is also characterized by loss of energy and pain in the legs, limbs and joints. It was given its identification as a result of the discoverer, Szent-Gyorgyi of Hungary, finding certain therapeutic qualities in paprika that cured a case of blood vessel bleeding. Another interesting reason for the selection of the letter "p" was the word "permeable." It was determined that this substance stabilized the permeability of blood vessels. The term refers to the ability of a liquid to pass through a structure without affecting it injuriously.

Result of deficiency. Lack of this substance in the blood apparently leads to a predisposition toward hemorrhage or bleeding where the blood vessels are thin and tiny, as in capillaries. Symptoms are swelling of tissues, pain in legs, limbs and joints, weakness of muscles generally, and easy tiring.

Availability. Natural vegetable juices, especially paprika juice. Also, the whole lemon contains a factor called citrine, having an effect similar to Vitamin P.

VITAMIN–CHOLINE

Value. Choline is said to be a Vitamin B complex vitamin. Technically, it is in its natural form a ptomaine found in the bile and suprarenal (above the kidney) gland extract. It is essential for proper functioning of the liver. Although made in the body through synthesis, it is not made in sufficient amounts to meet the needs of most higher animals. It must therefore be supplied in food. Chole is the Greek word for bile and this explains the use of the name choline. It meets the requirements for classification as a vitamin and is considered essential for growth and for the prevention of fatty livers. It retains its value despite exposure to heat and is well preserved in dried foods over long periods.

In addition to participating in the transport and metabolism of fats, it plays a role in the normal functioning of nerves and is important in the metabolism process, especially in the synthesis of some proteins.

Result of deficiency. A choline deficiency may result in fatty livers with subsequent poor growth, edema, impaired cardiovascular system, and hemorrhagic conditions in the kidneys, heart muscles and adrenal glands (the glands over each kidney).

Availability. It is available in liberal quantities in egg yolk, whole grains, legumes, meats of all kinds, and wheat germ. Vegetables and milk have some choline content but most other foods, including fruits, have little or no choline.

VITAMIN—PANTOTHENIC ACID

Value. This vitamin is needed for the proper functioning of the entire digestive system, especially by the adrenal gland. This member of the B-vitamin family is also known as calcium pantothenate and is generally recognized as essential for growth. Food processing has often removed this vitamin from the final food product placed on the store shelves.

Result of deficiency. When this vitamin is lacking or deficient in the body, there is reason to believe that this may be a factor in causing rheumatoid arthritis, grey hair, skin diseases, constipation, rough skin, granulation of the eyelids, digestive disorders and damage to the adrenal glands. This vitamin has been deemed essential to adequate functioning of the brain, and a lack of it may cause profound mental depression. Deficiency in this vitamin may prevent conception in the female or children born may be seriously deformed or mentally deficient. Muscular tissue requires an abundant supply of this vitamin and it must be remembered that the heart is a muscle. Other studies indicate an increase in the lifespan of 19 percent when there is plentiful pantothenic acid in the diet. At least 3 mg; daily is recommended.

Availability. This vitamin is found naturally in royal jelly honey, human milk, egg yolk, wheat bran, brewer's yeast, broccoli, molasses, peanuts, liver, kidney and in nearly all vegetable tissue. It's discoverer, Dr. Roger J. Williams, reports that perhaps the richest source is the ovary of the codfish. One report states that this valuable vitamin has been synthesized and that synthetic pantothenic acid obtains effective results.

PART II
ANALYSIS OF NUTRITIVE BENEFITS OF FRUITS, VEGETABLES, NUTS AND SEEDS

HOW TO USE THIS SECTION
OF FRUITS, VEGETABLES, NUTS AND SEEDS
FOR THE HEALTH INFORMATION YOU WANT

Alphabetical arrangement. All of the fruits, vegetables, nuts and seeds in this encyclopedia have been arranged in *alphabetical order* so they can be more easily located. To have arranged them in categories would have created confusion. The tomato, for example, is technically the fruit of a plant, but it is commonly known as a vegetable. To learn about the tomato one need only to find it's place in the alphabetical listing, without concern as to its technical category.

Quantities expressed in one hundred grams. Throughout the encyclopedia section, there are references to quantities of grams (gm) and milligrams (mg). For the foods listed here, the quantity is usually one cup, although of course a cup of raisins would be heavier than a cup of chopped celery. The controlling weight is one hundred grams, which is equivalent to 3 1/2 ounces avoirdupois. Thus, for example, almonds contain 18.6 gm. of protein per 100 gm., which means that in an ordinary serving of almonds of approximately 3 1/2 ounces there would be 18.6 grams of protein. In a similar manner, almonds contain 254 milligrams of calcium in 100 grams which, again, is the quantity of the usual individual serving.

Calories. Technically, a calory is the amount of heat necessary to raise the temperature of one kilogram of water from zero to 1° Centigrade. As a standard of measurement, an adult moving about during the day but not doing muscular work probably uses 2,450 calories, while a man doing hard muscular labor may use 5,500 calories. For comparison, one serving of almonds (100 grams) would provide an individual with 597 calories. It is desirable to consume sufficient food to provide sufficient calories for the day's work or activity. Of course, a variety of food is necessary in order to provide the necessary vitamins, minerals and other nutrients necessary.

Minerals. The minerals for each food item are shown in milligrams (mg). A milligram is one thousandth of a gram (gm). A milligram may not appear to be very much, but one must remember that the total mineral weight of the body is relatively low. Calcium, for example, comprises only 1.5 percent of the human body. Other percentages are: phosphorus, 1.0 percent; potassium, 0.35 percent; sulfur, 0.15 percent; chlorine, 0.15 percent; magnesium, 0.05 percent; iron, 0.04 percent; iodine, 0.00004 percent, and there are only tiny traces of copper, manganese, zinc, fluorine, silicon, cobalt, aluminum, arsenic and nickel. Twenty to thirty grams of mineral salts are excreted daily by an adult man under normal conditions, and the lost minerals need to be replaced daily in the food intake.

Carbohydrates and fat: The items in the encyclopedia section show the carbohydrate and fat content of each item in grams. As indicated in the previous section, both carbohydrates and fat are necessary to provide energy and heat. In addition, fat protects the body from rapid cooling and serves as a protective covering for delicate organs such as the eye and kidneys.

Vitamins: For Vitamin A, the measurement is in International Units (I.U.) per one hundred grams. Scientists around the world are not entirely in agreement as to how much carotene (vegetable pigment converted in the liver by the enzyme carotenase into Vitamin A) is equivalent to an International Unit of Vitamin A. The units shown in the encyclopedia for Vitamin A are on the basis of one I.U. of Vitamin A being equal to 0.6 microgram of beta carotene and 1.2 micrograms of other carotenes having Vitamin A activity. A microgram is one-millionth part of a gram. As an example, carrots are shown having carotene as 12,000 I.U. per 100 grams. When this number of I.U. is multiplied by 1.2 micrograms, the result is 14,400 micrograms. Inasmuch as it would take 1,000,000 micrograms to equal one gram, we can see that the amount of Vitamin A that the body receives by consuming 100 grams of carrots is small indeed. This is one good reason why so many people will take fruits and vegetables in juice form, enabling them to ingest many more vitamins into their systems.

ACEROLA CHERRY

Botanical information: The acerola cherry is the fruit of the *malphighia punici jolia* tree.

Nutritive values:

Vitamin B: Thiamine   .02   mg.;
   Riboflavin   .06   mg.; Niacin   4
   mg.
Vitamin C: 1300 mg.
Proteins: .4 gm.
Calories: 28

Fat: .3 gm.
Carbohydrates: 6.8 gm.
Calcium: 12 mg.
Iron: .2 mg.
Phosphorus: 11 mg.

Reported health benefits: The high Vitamin C content of this fruit makes the cherry excellent for supplying the body with the ascorbic acid needed for maintenance of good health. It has been found helpful for tender or painful swelling of the joints, loss of appetite, loss of weight, irritable temper, poor complexion, loss of energy, irregular heart action, rapid respiration, reduced hemoglobin, cataracts and hemorrhages.

Preparation: The raw acerola cherries are rather difficult to obtain but they are available in wafer form or in juice form at the markets.

ACORN

Botanical information: The fruit of the oak tree *(Quercus)*

Nutritive values: Although the exact amounts of the various nutrients are not available, the acorn is reported to be rich in Vitamin A, the B-Complex vitamins, unsaturated fatty acids and tannin.

Reported health benefits: The high oil and starch content of the acorn makes it very nutritious and is reported to be easily digested. It is also recommended for the skin, eyes and nerves. The tannin content helps to combat chronic diarrhea.

Preparation: With the modern kitchen equipment we now have, acorn meal can be prepared easily at home. After husking the acorns, they should be ground in a meal or food chopper. Then mix the meal with hot water and pour into a jelly bag, rinsing thoroughly until all the water-soluble tannin is removed. After washing, the wet meal is spread out to dry and is then parched in the oven.

The acorn meal may be used in the same way as corn meal in the baking of breads and muffins. The best meal is made from the acorns of the white oak trees, as the black oaks are quite bitter.

ALMONDS

Botanical information: The nut-like stone of the fruit of the almond tree of the rose family *Amygdalus communis.*

Nutritive values:

Vitamins: Contains B_1 (Thiamine) 0.25 mg.; B_2 (Riboflavin) 0.67 mg.; Niacin 4.6 mg.

Mineral content: Contains calcium (254 mg.), iron (4.4 mg.) and phosphorus (475 mg.).

Carbohydrates and fat: 19.6 gm. and 54.1 gm. respectively.

Protein: 18.6 gm. per 100 gm.

Calories: 597 per 100 gm.

Almond nuts also contain potassium, magnesium and phosphates, the latter being especially valuable for nourishing the nerve cells.

Reported health benefits: Almonds and almond butter are very nourishing foods and are recognized as muscle and body builders. The high fat, carbohydrate and protein content make it an ideal food for strengthening the body when there is no need to worry about the increase in the supply of fat. The content of calcium makes it valuable for the teeth and bones.

Preparation: Almonds are delicious as substitutes for candy or other sweets, but these nuts are also popular for baking in cookies, cakes and breads, as well as in fruit and vegetable salads.

A healthy and delicious fruit and vegetable salad with almonds is prepared by combining two cups of grapefruit segments with one-half cup of chopped dates and a cup of shredded almonds. An attractive appearance is made by arranging the ingredients on lettuce leaves, with green pepper rings spread over the leaves and with the grapefruit and dates in equal proportions placed on the pepper rings, and the shredded almonds sprinkled over all. There can be all kinds of variations, substituting oranges or tangerines for the grapefruit or having some portions of each, or substituting figs for the dates or having both of these ingredients. Watercress could be substituted for the lettuce and perhaps slices of avocado or other fruits such as apples or pears added or substituted, depending upon what is available or more economical. Instead of shredding the almonds, they may be used in whole form.

APPLE

Botanical information: The apple is the fruit of the tree *Malus malus* of the family *Pomaceae.*

Nutritive values:

Vitamin A: 900 I.U. per 100 gm.

Vitamin B: Thiamine .07 mg.; Riboflavin .03 mg.; Niacin .2 mg.

Vitamin C: 5 mg.

Vitamin G: Amount uncertain.

Protein: .3 gm.

Calories: 58

Fat: .4 gm.

Carbohydrates: 14.9 gm.

Calcium: 6 mg.

Iron: .3 mg.

Phosphorus: 10 mg.

Potassium: 130 mg.

Reported health benefits: The apple stimulates all body secretions and is well known not only as a food but as a beverage (apple juice), health tonic, medicine, cosmetic and bowel regulator all in one. The large variety of minerals and vitamins strengthens the blood. Apples also contain malic and tartaric acids, which help prevent disturbances of the liver and digestion in general. It has been reported that where unsweetened apple cider is used as a beverage the formation of kidney stones is unknown. The low acidity of the apples stimulates salivary flow and thus helps to remove debris from the teeth and stimulates gum tissues. Studies also indicate that eating apples daily will reduce skin diseases, arthritis, and various lung and asthma problems. Apples are said to prevent emotional upsets, tension and headaches. The rind or peel of the apple contains pectin, which helps to remove noxious substances from the system by supplying galacturonic acid. The pectin helps to prevent protein matter in the intestines from spoiling.

Apples have also been recommended for obesity correction, skin eruption, poor complexion, inflammation of the bladder, gonorrhea, anemia, tuberculosis, neuritis, insomnia, catarrh, gall stones, worms, halitosis and pyorrhea.

Preparation: Every effort should be made to avoid fruit sprayed with poisonous pesticides. The best way to eat them is to wash them and eat them unpeeled in order to avoid losing the nutrients and beneficial substances that are part of the skin.

In addition to the apple juice drink, an apple tea is popular with many people and it is said that this will cleanse the urinary tract and help various diseases of the male and female reproductive organs. The apples are sliced with the peeling left on. The slices are placed in a pan lined with white paper and the pan is then placed in a moderate oven (350°F) with the oven door left open. When the slices are thoroughly dried, the oven door should be closed and the apples roasted until they turn a dark brown color. The slices are then stored in a dry place until needed. The tea is made the same as other tea. The slices are placed in a cup and hot water poured over it, and steeping goes on for about ten minutes before there has been sufficient absorption of the ingredients of the apple.

There is actually an unlimited number of ways of preparing apples. They are often cut into slices and served with other fruit in a salad or they are included in cake, cookie and pie recipes.

A delicious apple pie pudding is made by slicing the apples, adding enough honey to sweeten and combining with a little lemon juice and sufficient water so all the ingredients will mix well. If desired, some graham cracker crumbs may be added. The mixture is then turned into an oiled baking dish and baked in a moderate oven (375° F) for thirty minutes or until the apples are tender.

APRICOT

Botanical information: The fruit of the tree *Prunus armeniaca.*

Nutritive values:

Vitamin A: 2,790 I.U. per 100 gm.   Fat: .1 gm.
Vitamin B: Thiamine .03 mg.;   Carbohydrates: 12.9 gm.
   Riboflavin .05 mg.; Niacin .8 mg.   Calcium: 16 mg.
Vitamin C: 7 mg.   Iron: .5 mg.
Protein: 1.0 gm.   Phosphorus: 23 mg.
Calories: 51   Potassium: 280 mg.

Reported health benefits: The high iron content and richness in minerals makes this fruit beneficial in cases of anemia, tuberculosis, asthma, bronchitis, catarrh, and toxemia or blood impurities. It is also excellent for diets designed to reduce weight and for the removal of skin pimples and diarrhea. Reports also indicate that it will help cases of constipation and will destroy intestinal worms. Other reports indicate that apricots will remove gall stones.

Preparation: Apricots are used in cake-making, breads, cookies, fillings, jams, pies, puddings, salads and stews. They are also eaten raw for an occasional snack.

A healthy and delicious pudding can be made by soaking one-half pound of apricots overnight and then stewing them until tender. One-half cup of honey is then added, and after mixing and bringing to a boil, pour the mixture into a casserole lined in the bottom and around the sides with toasted whole wheat bread slices. Bake with raisins and sprinkle with cinnamon. Cover the casserole, allow to cool gradually and serve. Where obesity is not a problem, the individual portions may be covered with some cream or whole milk.

A delicious and nourishing fruit salad is made by shredding two cups of lettuce and placing halves of apricots, peaches and pears alternately in circles over the lettuce. Some yogurt may be dropped over the salad for additional good taste and nourishment.

ARTICHOKE

Botanical information: Thistle-like plant, *Cynara scolymus,* of the aster family.

Nutritive values:

Vitamin A: 150 I.U. per 100 gm.

Vitamin B: Thiamine 150 mg.;
Riboflavin, trace; Niacin .7 mg.

Vitamin C: 8 mg.

Protein: 2 gm.

Calories: 44

Fat: trace

Carbohydrates: 10 gm.

Calcium: 50 mg.

Iron: 1.3

Phosphorus: 69 mg.

Potassium: 300 mg.

Reported health benefits: The juice of the leaves is reportedly a powerful diuretic (kidney stimulant) and also effective in liver ailments and for dropsy. Other reports indicate that the artichoke is valuable for anemia, excessive acidity, diarrhea, rheumatism, halitosis or bad breath, obesity, neuritis, and glandular disorders.

Preparation: They are best prepared by steaming them only long enough for softening. The leaves are usually picked off, one at a time, and drawn through the front teeth for scraping off the tender part. The leaf is held by the tip and if dietary restrictions do not forbid the use of butter, the end of the leaf may be dipped into melted butter for additional flavoring. After all the leaves are removed, the "hairy" part above the center core is removed and the delicious center core or "heart" may be eaten with a fork.

A nourishing artichoke omelet may be made by adding to the beaten eggs before placing them into the omelet pan several artichoke "hearts" equal in number to the number of eggs in the omelet. The hearts should be first prepared by cooking until soft and chopped into several pieces. For additional flavoring and health value, add a finely chopped clove of garlic and several tablespoons of finely chopped onion. Two tablespoons of olive oil may be added for additional flavor and nourishment to the egg mixture before cooking the omelet.

The artichoke leaves and hearts are excellent for serving with a dish of vegetables for a luncheon vegetable treat.

ASPARAGUS

Botanical information: The tender, succulent shoots of *Asparagus officinalis,* cut when projecting a little above the ground.

Nutritive values:

Vitamin A: 1,000 I.U. per gm.

Vitamin B: Thiamine .16 mg.;
Riboflavin .19 mg.; Niacin 1.4 mg.

Fat: .2 gm.

Carbohydrates: 3.9 gm.

Calcium: 21 mg.

Iron: .9 mg.

Vitamin C: 33 mg.   Phosphorus: 62 mg.
Protein: 2.2 gm.   Potassium: 130 mg.
Calories: 82

Reported health benefits: It has been reported that the juice of the asparagus helps to break up oxalic acid crystals in the kidneys and throughout the muscular system, thereby making asparagus juice good for rheumatism, neuritis, arthritis and similar ailments.

Preparation: The most common method of preparation is to tie the asparagus into bundles, with perhaps ten stalks to a bundle. The bundles are then placed in a pot of water with the tips up and the thick stalk-ends at the bottom. Add only enough water to cover the thick parts of the stalks and cook for ten minutes or until stalks are tender. Then arrange the bundles so the tips are covered with water and cook for five minutes longer. They may then be served, sprinkling with pepper. Salt may be used if not contrary to diet restrictions. However, ordinary table salt should be avoided and salt in natural form as sea salt should be used when available.

To prepare asparagus with scrambled eggs, first cook the asparagus tips, add some unbeaten eggs and mix together. Add some seasoning, and after melting some butter in a frying pan, add the eggs with the asparagus and cook over a slow fire, stirring constantly until the eggs are set solid. Serve on hot, buttered whole wheat toast.

A tempting vegetable salad is made by spreading out the asparagus tips as though radiating from the hub of a wheel. Various other vegetables are spread around the plate such as tomatoes, celery, lettuce and cucumbers, sliced and cut to appropriate sizes.

AVOCADO

Botanical information: The fruit of the tree *Persea persea* of the laurel family.

Nutritive values:

Vitamin A: 290 I.U. per 100 gm.   Fat: 26.4 gm.
Vitamin B: Thiamine 290 mg.;   Carbohydrates: 5.1 gm.
   Riboflavin .13 mg.; Niacin 1.1   Calcium: 10 mg.
   mg.   Iron: .6 mg.
Vitamin C: 16 mg.   Phosphorus: 38 mg.
Protein: 1.7 gm.   Potassium: 600 mg.
Calories: 245

Reported health benefits: This nourishing and delicious food has been recommended for malnutrition because of the plentiful supply of vitamins and minerals. It has a smooth texture and is therefore a food that may be readily taken by ulcer sufferers. In addition, the avocado has been recommended for inflamed conditions of the mucous membrane, particularly of the small intestines and the colon. The richness of nutrients has apparently made it helpful for cases of male impotency and it is also reported as helpful for cases of constipation, insomnia and nervousness.

Preparation: Avocado is delicious itself as a snack but it can also be prepared in numerous ways.

An unusual and delicious preparation is to take an avocado or two and make a cut lengthwise, removing the seed and replacing the area of the seed with chopped celery mixed with salmon or cheese, or almost any other food combinations.

The avocado is so versatile that it may be used either as a fruit salad or as part of a vegetable salad. In fact, there may be a combination of both, such as alternate slices of avocado, grapefruit and tomato. The varieties are innumerable. In all salads, cottage cheese should not be overlooked as an ingredient.

BAMBOO SHOOTS

Botanical information: The genus *Bambusa.*

Nutritive values:

Vitamin A: 20 I.U. per 100 grams	Fat: .3 gm.
Vitamin B: Thiamine .15 mg.;	Carbohydrates: 5.2 gm.
Riboflavin .07 mg.; Niacin .6 mg.	Calcium: 13 mg.
Vitamin C: 4 mg.	Iron: .5 mg.
Protein: 2.6 gm.	Phosphorus: 59 mg.
Calories: 27	

Reported health benefits: Bamboo shoots have been recommended in cases of constipation, worms, obesity, high blood pressure, and toxemia (internal poisoning).

Preparation: The tender bamboo shoots are edible raw or they may be softened by boiling them for about ten minutes. The young shoots are the only edible parts of the bamboo.

BANANA

Botanical information: The banana is the fruit of the banana plant *Musa sapientum.*

Nutritive values:

Vitamin A: 430 I.U. per 100 gm.   Fat: .2 gm.
Vitamin B: Thiamine .04 mg.;   Carbohydrates: 23 gm.
   Riboflavin .05 mg.; Niacin .7 mg.   Calcium: 8 mg.
Vitamin C: 10 mg.   Iron: .6 mg.
Protein: 1.2 gm.   Phosphorus: 28 mg.
Calories: 88   Potassium: 260 mg.

Reported health benefits: When ripe, usually indicated by the presence of spots, bananas are not only used as a snack treat but are valuable for various ailments, such as stomach ulcers, colitis, diarrhea, hemorrhoids, and for general energy. Reports indicate that the inner surface of the banana skin may be applied directly to burns or boils for the healing effect.

Preparation: There are many ways of preparing bananas aside from merely peeling them and eating them, which is the most popular way. They can be baked, included in cake, cookie and bread recipes, used in ice cream, puddings and pies, and made into fruit salads.

Sweet potatoes and bananas may be combined and baked in a casserole to make a delicious side dish for the main meal. Take some bananas and sweet potatoes in the proportion of twice as many potatoes as bananas. Cook the potatoes until soft and slice them to 1/4 inch thickness. Peel and slice the bananas, arranging the potatoes and bananas in alternate layers in a greased casserole dish, sprinkling honey or brown sugar over each layer. Repeat the building of the layers until they reach the height of the casserole. Cinnamon may be added over each layer for additional flavor. Add some water to the casserole (preferably from the water used to boil the potatoes) sufficient to thoroughly moisten all of the contents, and bake in a hot oven of 400°F for twenty-five minutes with the casserole covered. After the time indicated, remove the cover and bake again until brown.

BARLEY

Botanical information: Barley is the grain of the cultivated grass of the genus *Hordeum*.

Nutritive values:

Vitamin B: Thiamine .12 mg.;   Fat: 1.0 gm.
   Riboflavin .08 mg.; Niacin 3.1   Carbohydrates: 78.8 gm.
   mg.   Calcium: 16 mg.

Protein: 8.2 gm.   Iron: 2.0 mg. (uncertain)
Calories: 349   Phosphorus: 189 mg.

Reported health benefits: Barley is highly regarded as a nutritious food, and for under-weight individuals this food will do much to increase body weight. It is also reported as mild and nutritious enough to help heal stomach ulcers and relieve diarrhea. It is said to help prevent tooth decay or loss of hair and is said to improve the condition of the nails of the hands and feet. Barley water has been found to be valuable in correcting cases of gravel stones and high fever. It may also be useful in asthma because of a substance, Hordenine, which relieves bronchial spasms.

Preparation: To prepare a good barley water drink, take two ounces of barley and boil it in three pints of water until the quantity of water is reduced to one-half the original amount. To make the drink more of a laxative nature, add two ounces of sliced figs. For additional flavoring and sweetening, add two ounces of raisins to the mixture. One-half ounce of licorice root may be added for additional flavoring.

An efficient way of preparing a good drink for bowel disorders is to tie a quantity of barley meal into a linen cloth and boil it for half an hour in some water. The liquid remaining is considered to be a good drink for bowel disorders.

In preparing barley as a breakfast cereal, use three to four cups of water to a cup of barley, preferably using the unpearled barley variety in order to retain the maximum amount of vitamins and minerals. For additional nourishment and flavor, raisins may be added during the cooking process and milk added when ready to serve. Honey may be used for additional sweetening.

BEANS, LIMA AND OTHER SPECIES

Botanical information: The bean is the seed of the plants of the bean family *Fabaceae*.

Nutritive values:

Vitamin A: 280 I.U. per 100 gm.   Fat: .8 gm.
Vitamin B: Thiamine .21 mg.;   Carbohydrates: 23.5 gm.
   Riboflavin .11 mg.; Niacin 1.4   Calcium: 63 mg.
   mg.   Iron: 2.3 mg.
Vitamin C: 32 mg.   Phosphorus: 158 mg.
Protein: 7.5 gm.   Potassium: 200 mg.
Calories: 128

Reported health benefits: Lima and butter beans have been found to be so rich in vitamins and minerals, especially in iron, that this food is considered a wonderful food for persons suffering from anemia. These beans are also highly recommended for other ailments where body building and muscular development is desirable, such as cases of emaciation, malnutrition, and tuberculosis. Beans have also been found helpful for persons suffering from hemorrhoids.

Preparation: Beans are usually prepared by washing, shelling, and then boiling for twenty to thirty minutes in an amount of water sufficient to cover the beans until tender. After cooking and draining, the water drained should be saved and either used as a cold drink or as stock for soups, as a large share of the mineral and vitamin content is absorbed by the water during the process of cooking. The beans may then be served as a side dish with the main meal.

A good recipe for bean soup, whether lima or otherwise, is to soak the beans overnight and drain the water. There will be little, if any, nourishment in this water, so it may be discarded. For serving from eight to ten persons, use two cups of lima beans, navy beans, black soybeans or black beans and cook in three quarts of water, adding a tablespoon of chopped onions, a tablespoon of chopped parsley, two cups of chopped celery, a cup of cut-up potatoes, two sliced hard-boiled eggs, one sliced lemon, two dashes of cayenne pepper, four tablespoons of butter, three cloves, one cut-up carrot, and a dash or two of pepper. Heat to boiling and cook over a slow heat until the potatoes are tender. From one-half to a cup of milk may be added just before serving.

Cooked lima beans are often used in a vegetable salad, placing the beans on lettuce leaves and adding slices of tomato and slices of hard-boiled egg. A good salad dressing can be made by combining one-half cup olive oil with one-quarter cup lemon juice and the juice of one tomato.

BEECHNUT

Botanical information: The beechnut is a small, triangular, edible nut of the beech tree, of the genus *Fagus*. It is found in temperate regions.

Nutritive values:

Protein: 19.4 gm. per 100 gm. Fat: 50.0 gm.
Calories: 568 Carbohydrates: 20.3 gm

Reported health benefits: The high protein and fat content makes this a good body-building food, especially for anemia victims. The large number of calories provide for considerable energy. The carbohydrates produce both heat and energy.

Preparation: As with other nuts, beechnuts may be eaten raw or ground.

BEETS, COMMON RED

Botanical information: The biennial herb *Beta vulgaris* of the goosefoot family. A fleshy and succulent root.

Nutritive values:

Vitamin A: 20 I.U. per 100 gm.

Vitamin B: Thiamine .02 mg.; Riboflavin .05 mg.; Niacin .4 mg.

Vitamin C: 10 mg.

Protein: 1.6 gm.

Calories: 42

Fat: .1 gm.

Carbohydrates: 9.6 gm.

Calcium: 27 mg.

Iron: 1.0 mg.

Phosphorus: 43 mg.

Reported health benefits: The blood-building nutrients in beets furnish excellent food for the red blood corpuscles. Beets have been recommended for headaches and toothaches as well as for inflammation of the kidneys and bladder, including bladder and kidney stone ailments. A special red beet therapy, consisting of consumption of approximately two pounds of raw, mashed beets daily, has been favorably reported for cases of leukemia and tumors. Red beets have also been reported valuable for cases of constipation, liver ailments (jaundice), dysentery (inflammation of intestines), skin disorders such as pimples, obesity, lumbago, anemia, nervousness, and menstruation problems.

Preparation: Beets may be shredded or cut into slices and served with other raw vegetables as a salad, or they may be ground and served as a side dish.

When beets are cooked to make them tender, they should be eaten without removal of the skins in order to avoid losing the nutrients in the skin and close to the skin.

A good dressing for spreading over raw beets is to spread some honey over the beets and other vegetables on the dish and sprinkle some lemon juice over all the vegetables.

A cooked beet soup is made by taking the beets and cutting them into cubes and also cutting in the same manner (known as dicing) a medium-sized onion. A small head of cabbage may be added to the soup, first shredding the cabbage into small pieces. Add one or two dashes of pepper to taste. Natural salt may be added if not restricted to a no-salt diet. Instead of cabbage other vegetables may be added, such as tomatoes, potatoes, carrots, green peppers, or other vegetables. Only a minimum amount of water should be added and cooking continued only until the vegetables are tender. If possible, a steam cooker should be used so that no water at all need be added.

BEET GREENS

Botanical information: The plant of the biennial herb *Reta vulgaris* of the goosefoot family. Edible greens are from the white, Sicilian or Swiss chard-beet.

Nutritive values:

Vitamin A: 6,700 I.U. per 100 gm.	Fat: .3 gm.
Vitamin B: Thiamine .08 mg.; Riboflavin .18 mg.; Niacin .4 mg.	Carbohydrates: 5.6 gm.
	Calcium: 118 mg.
Vitamin C: 34 mg.	Iron: 3.2 mg.
Protein: 2.0 gm.	Phosphorus: 45 mg.
Calories: 27	Potassium: 332 mg.

Reported health benefits: Beet greens, especially the tops of the red beets, are richer than spinach in iron and other minerals. They are reported to help cases of anemia, constipation, poor appetite, dysentery (inflammation of mucous membrane of the intestines), pimples and other skin disorders, gas, gout, tumors, tonsilitis, obesity, tuberculosis and gonorrhea. There is a high oxalic acid content and an excess should be avoided.

Preparation: To cook the tops of beets, first discard the wilted leaves and remove the roots, which of course have special value. (See Beets, common red.) Wash quickly in warm water (not hot) to remove sand and soil, then wash several times in cold water. Place in saucepan without adding water and cover tightly to prevent escape of steam. Cook over low heat for ten to fifteen minutes. When serving, sprinkle with herbs and spices for flavoring.

Beet greens may also be prepared with beet roots. If possible, select young beets, wash the tops, and steam in one-half cup water until tender. Cut the tops and season with sweet butter. Steam the beets until they are tender and place in cold water; remove the skin if you must. From the health point of view the skins are good for you, as they contain minerals that are beneficial. Serve the greens in a large bowl and top the greens with buttered beets. Hard-boiled eggs may be sliced and placed around the edge of the bowl, garnishing with sections of lemon.

BLACKBERRY

Botanical information: A variety of small succulent fruit, with the seeds in a juicy pulp. The species is *Rubus* of the rose family, *Rosaceae.*
Nutritive values:

Vitamin A: 200 I.U. per 100 gm.

Vitamin B: Thiamine .04 mg.; Riboflavin .04 mg.; Niacin .4 mg.

Vitamin C: 21 mg.

Protein: 1.2 gm.

Calories: 57

Fat: 1.0 gm.

Carbohydrates: 12.5 gm.

Calcium: 32 mg.

Iron: .9 mg.

Phosphorus: 32 mg.

Reported health benefits: Blackberries are reported to be valuable as a general tonic and blood cleanser. They have been recommended for constipation, anemia, obesity, weak kidneys, rheumatism, arthritis, gout, pimples and other skin problems, and diarrhea. In addition, they are reported as helpful for catarrh or running of mucus from the sinuses and for dysentery, inflammation of the intestines. The unripe berries are said to be valuable to treat hemorrhages and to be helpful for menstrual cramps. In addition, the leaves of the blackberry may be used for treatment of sore throat, boiling water being poured over the leaves and the water then allowed to cool until comfortable for gargling.

Preparation: Blackberries are commonly used as a dessert dish after the main meal, perhaps sprinkled with honey for extra flavoring.

A good recipe for blackberry pudding is to add one beaten egg to each cup of blackberries together with one-half cup milk, one-half cup honey, and a teaspoon of baking powder. A cup of whole wheat flour is added to the mixture, with perhaps one-half cup of raisins. After thorough mixing it is poured into a greased pan, covered and baked in a moderate oven (350°F) for about thirty minutes or until browned.

BLUEBERRY

Botanical information: The fruit of a shrub of the species of *Vaccinium.*

Nutritive values:

Vitamin A: 280 I.U. per 100 gm.   Fat: .6 gm.
Vitamin B: Thiamine .02 mg.;   Carbohydrates: 15.1 gm.
  Riboflavin .02 mg.; Niacin .3 mg.   Calcium: 16 mg.
Vitamin C: 16 mg.   Iron: .8 mg.
Protein: .6 gm.   Phosphorus: 13 mg.
Calories: 61

Reported health benefits: Blueberries are known as blood cleansers and for antiseptic use. They are recommended for anemia, constipation, diarrhea, obesity, menstrual disorders and poor skin complexion. The antiseptic value of blueberries is apparently what helps conditions of inflammation of the intestines known as dysentery, which in turn contributes to the condition of diarrhea.

Preparation: In addition to partaking of blueberries as a side dish or dessert as part of a meal, a very popular food delicacy is the blueberry muffin. By making a few substitutions to eliminate the white sugar and white flour from the recipe, a fairly healthy product can be produced. For about a dozen muffins, take two cups of whole wheat flour and mix with four teaspoons of baking powder and one-half teaspoon of salt, although salt should be omitted if anyone has high blood pressure and/or is on a salt-free diet. One egg is then beaten into a cup of milk and 1/4 cup of honey, in lieu of sugar. One-quarter cup of butter, peanut oil or other pure vegetable oil should then be added to the liquids and beaten well. The mixtures are then combined after first adding a cup of blueberries to the dry ingredients. There is only a small amount of mixing, just enough so that the flour becomes damp. If not mixed excessively, the muffins will be of a fine texture; otherwise, they may fall flat. The mixture is poured into muffin pans only 2/3 full and baked in an oven previously heated to 400°F for twenty-five minutes.

BRAZIL NUTS

Botanical information: The edible seed of a tall South American tree *Bertholletia excelsa* of the family *Lecythidaceae.*

Nutritive values:

Vitamin A: Only a trace per 100 gm.   Carbohydrates: 11.0 gm.
Vitamin B: Thiamine .08 mg.;   Calcium: 186 mg.
  Riboflavin none; Niacin none   Iron: 3.4 mg.
Protein: 14.4 gm.   Phosphorus: 693 mg.

Calories: 646   Potassium: 660 mg.
Fat: 65.9 gm.

Reported health benefits: Brazil nuts and the butter made from the nuts is a very nourishing food. It is especially good for muscular workers, and the richness of calcium makes this a good food for the teeth and bones. These nuts are also recommended for all-round nutrition deficiencies for the relief of malnutrition.

Preparation: They may be eaten as a confection; however, there are endless possibilities for the use of Brazil nuts in cakes, cookies, pies, puddings, and in combination with other foods of every variety.

One example is baking apples with the use of Brazil nuts in the center of the apple instead of raisins, bananas, honey, or other fruits or jellies.

BREADFRUIT

Botanical information: The fruit of the tree *artocarpus commun,* originally grown in the South Seas, now cultivated in the West Indies.

Nutritive values:

Vitamin A: 40 I.U. per 100 gm   Fat: .3 gm.
Vitamin B: Thiamine .11 mg.;   Carbohydrates: 26.2 gm.
    Riboflavin .03 mg.; Niacin .9 mg.   Calcium: 33 mg.
Vitamin C: 29 mg.   Iron: 1.2 mg.
Protein: 1.7 gm.   Phosphorus: 32 mg.
Calories: 103

Reported health benefits: One of the most nourishing starchy foods of the South Seas. An excellent general body builder, especially recommended for muscular workers.

Preparation: When mature, the breadfruit is about the size of a large grapefruit. It is generally boiled and eaten as one would eat a potato.

BROCCOLI

Botanical information: Broccoli is a variety of cabbage but is hardier. The botanical name is *Brassica oleracea botrytis.*

Nutritive values:

Vitamin A: 3,500 I.U. per 100 gm.   Fat: .2 gm.

Vitamin B: Thiamine .10 mg.;   Carbohydrates: 5.5 gm.
   Riboflavin .21 mg.; Niacin 1.1   Calcium: 130 mg.
   mg.   Iron: 1.3 mg.
Vitamin C: 118 mg. Also contains   Phosphorus: 76 mg.
   Vitamins E and K.   Potassium: 270 mg.
Protein: 3.3 gm.
Calories: 29

Reported health benefits: Broccoli is an excellent food for reducing overweight (obesity) and for constipation, toxemia, neuritis, high blood pressure, and weak glands involved in digestion of foods.

Preparation: After washing the broccoli, the thick heads may be split into two parts and the broccoli cooked with ends down and heads out of water for ten to twenty minutes, with the pot uncovered. After this period of time, all of the broccoli should be cooked under water for five minutes. Season with some herbs or spices when ready to serve.

BRUSSELS SPROUTS

Botanical information: *Brassica oleracea,* a variety of cabbage known as *bullata gemmifera* with blistered leaves and stems covered with heads.

Nutritive values:

Vitamin A: 400 I.U. per 100 gm.   Fat: .5 gm.
Vitamin B: .08 mg.   Carbohydrates: 8.9 gm.
Vitamin C: 94 mg.   Calcium: 34 mg.
Protein: 4.4 gm.   Iron: 1.3 mg.
Calories: 47   Phosphorus: 78 mg.
                                    Potassium: 307 mg.

Reported health benefits: This is reported to be a good general tonic food and recommended for catarrh, obesity, acidosis, constipation, and hardening of the arteries. This vegetable is also recommended for bleeding gums.

Preparation: The wilted leaves are removed from the sprouts, after which they are washed and allowed to stand in cold water for fifteen minutes. They are then placed in a pan and sufficient boiling water is poured over the sprouts to cover them. They are then cooked without a cover for from ten to twenty minutes. Spices should be added for extra taste and flavor.

BUTTERNUT

Botanical information: Also known as white walnut, this edible oily nut is from an American tree of the family *Juglans cinerea.*

Nutritive values:

Protein: 23.7 gm. per 100 gm.
Calories: 629

Fat: 61.2 gm.
Carbohydrates: 8.4 gm.
Iron: 6.8 mg.

Reported health benefits: The high protein and fat content, together with the large number of calories, makes this a good body-building food.

Preparation: They may be eaten raw or ground into a butter-like spread.

CABBAGE

Botanical information: *Brassica oleracea,* usually compact and globular form.

Nutritive values:

Vitamin A: 80 I.U. per 100 gm.
Vitamin B: Thiamine .06 mg.;
Riboflavin .05 mg.; Niacin .3 mg.
Vitamin C: 50 mg.
Protein: 1.4 gm.
Calories: 24

Fat: .2 gm.
Carbohydrates: 5.3 gm.
Calcium: 46 mg.
Iron: .5 mg.
Phosphorus: 31 mg.
Potassium: 140 mg.

Reported health benefits: The common cabbage has been highly recommended as a muscle builder, blood cleanser and eye strengthener. It has also been recommended for the teeth, gums, hair, nails, and bones, as well as for asthma, tuberculosis, gout, constipation, kidney and bladder disorders, obesity, diabetes, lumbago, and for improvement of the skin. Fresh raw cabbage juice has been acclaimed for alleviating stomach ulcers. It is an excellent iron tonic for cases where there is an iron deficiency. In addition to the foregoing listed vitamins and minerals, cabbage contains chlorine and sulphur, which help to cleanse the mucous membrane of the stomach and intestines. Many years ago, cabbage was commonly used for headaches, colic, deafness, insomnia and ulcers.

Preparation: Cabbage, red or white, should be eaten raw for best results.

The fresh juice drink is best for most effective value. The outer leaves have an abundant supply of calcium and should not be discarded. In addition, when cabbage is cut, slawed or shredded, much of the Vitamin C content is lost due to exposure to the air.

A healthy and delicious salad is made by shredding a cabbage and placing it on a salad dish with sliced apples.

Cabbage is cooked by first cutting a cabbage head into eight sections or into quarters. The pieces are then placed in a pan and covered with boiling water, then cooked, uncovered, until tender. Depending upon whether the cabbage is young or old, it will take from ten to twenty minutes for the cabbage to cook. Season with spices and serve.

A fairly complete meal can be made by arranging sections of cabbage in a baking dish on which some pure vegetable oil has been applied. Depending upon the quantity of cabbage and the size of the dish, several eggs are combined with milk on the basis of one cup of milk to an egg and then poured over the cabbage. Spices are then sprinkled over the entire dish, which is then placed in a pan of hot water and placed in a moderate oven of 350°F for 40 minutes or until the mixture of eggs and milk is firm. A cup of stewed tomatoes may be substituted for the milk and a tablespoon of minced (cut) onion may be added to the eggs and milk for additional taste and flavoring. When ready to serve, the food may be sprinkled with lemon juice for additional flavoring.

A nourishing cabbage combination is shredding the cabbage and adding it to scalded milk in a quantity sufficient to be covered by the milk. The cabbage is stirred thoroughly and then cooked slowly over a low flame for approximately fifteen to twenty minutes, stirring occasionally. Season with various herbs and spices to suit the taste.

CANTALOUPE

Botanical information: The cantaloupe is a variety of muskmelon, with a yellowish or pale-green skin and reddish flesh. Botanical name is *Cucumis melo.*

Nutritive values:

Vitamin A: 3,420 I.U. per 100 gm.   Fat: .2 gm.
Vitamin B: Thiamine .05 mg.;   Carbohydrates: 4.6 gm.
    Riboflavin .04 mg.; Niacin .5 mg.   Calcium: 17 mg.
Vitamin C: 33 mg.   Iron: .4 mg.

Protein: .6 gm. Phosphorus: 16 mg.
Calories: 20 Potassium: 242 mg.

Reported health benefits: The variety of vitamins, proteins and minerals in cantaloupes and other melons makes this fruit an excellent food. Cantaloupe has been recommended for cases where there is fever, high blood pressure, obesity, rheumatism, arthritis, disorders of the kidney and bladder, constipation, abdominal and stomach gas, skin diseases and blood deficiencies.

Preparation: The most popular method of consuming cantaloupe is merely scooping out the delicious meat from half of a cantaloupe after removal of the seeds. They are also popular with fruit salads, usually cut into slices and sometimes cut out with a special cutter in the form of small balls. An excellent combination is to prepare a mixture of cantaloupe with cherries and pineapple placed over some green vegetables, such as lettuce.

CARAMBOLA

Botanical information: Acid pulpy fruit of the tropical tree *averrhoa carambola.*
Nutritive values:

Vitamin A: 1200 I.U. per 100 gm. Fat: .5 gm.
Vitamin B: Thiamine .04 mg.; Carbohydrates: 8.0 gm.
  Riboflavin .02 mg.; Niacin .3 mg. Calcium: 4 mg.
Vitamin C: 35 mg. Iron: 1.5 mg.
Protein: .7 gm. Phosphorus: 17 mg.
Calories: 35

Reported health benefits: This delicious, exotic tropical fruit contains so many vitamins and minerals that it should be a great help in maintaining good health for those lucky people able to obtain it.

Preparation: It may be eaten raw or cut and sliced into portions for a fruit and/or vegetable salad.

CAROB

Botanical information: The fruit of an evergreen tree, *Ceratonia siliqua,* indigenous in the Mediterranean region.

Nutritive values: Carob is an excellent, well-balanced food, rich in Vitamins A and B-complex. It also contains valuable minerals, especially calcium and phosphorus for healthy teeth and bones, iron and copper for good red blood, and magnesium. It also is a good source of proteins and carbohydrates.

Reported health benefits: Aside from the general health benefits derived from the nutrients contained in carob, the flour made from the pod is also recommended as an effective medicine in cases of "non-specific" diarrheas—those caused by something other than a definite bacteria or disease. It has also been used successfully as an addition to the formula of babies who have not been able to keep any food in their stomachs.

Preparation: Carob flour is the fruit of the carob tree that has been finely ground, and is used as a replacement for cocoa, chocolate, and to some extent sugar. It may be purchased in flour form and used for home baking, or you may buy any of the carob products ready-made, such as delicious cookies, cakes and healthful candies.

CARROT

Botanical information: A variety of *Daucus carota.*

Nutritive values:

Vitamin A: 12,000 I.U. per 100 gm.	Fat: 0.3 gm,
Vitamin B: Thiamine .06 mg.; Riboflavin .06 mg.; Niacin .5 mg.	Carbohydrates: 9.3 gm.
	Calcium: 39 mg.
Vitamin C: 5 mg.	Iron: .8 mg.
Carrots also contain Vitamins D, E, G and K.	Phosphorus: 37 mg.
Protein: 1.2 gm.	
Calories: 42	

Reported health benefits: Carrots taken whole or as juice have been reported as valuable for cases of obesity, toxemia (poisoning of the blood), constipation, asthma, poor complexion, poor teeth (including pyorrhea), insomnia, high blood pressure, neurasthenia (nervous strain due to overwork), inflamed kidneys and bladder, colitis (inflammation of the colon), catarrh (discharge from mucous membrane), improves appearance of hair and nails, helps improve eyesight, corrects dropsy (excessive accumulation of fluid in body cavities), ends painful urination, increases menstrual flow, and helps to keep the skin healthy. As fresh carrots are an important source of Vitamin A, individuals deficient in this vitamin may be suffering from colds, due to the tendency of the cells of the skin and mucous membrane to dry up and become horny-like when deprived of this vitamin. This deficiency may cause the liver, kidneys and other glands, including the genital organs, to suffer. One symptom of lack of this vitamin is a loss of ability to smell. Another symptom is diarrhea. In addition, other glands affected are the thyroid, the pituitary (master gland in the cranium, attached to the base of the brain), and perhaps other glands and organs.

Carrot juice has been recommended for relief of peptic ulcers. The juice, taken in ample quantities, is also reported to prevent bodily infections, and is said to be valuable for the adrenal glands (the small glands situated above each kidney). Dr. N.W. Walker has reported that this juice will prevent infections of the eyes, throat, tonsils, the sinus area, and the lungs and lung passages. This juice has also been recommended for nursing mothers, to enhance the quality of their breast milk.

Preparation: Nutritionists generally agree that the greatest value of a food is preserved when it is eaten raw. Thus, carrots served with a salad or as raw carrot juice and served in a glass are probably the healthiest form of partaking of this food item.

Shredded carrots seem to have more food value than eating the whole carrot, tests showing that more of the carotene is absorbed into the body and is then converted into Vitamin A when the carrot is shredded or juiced than when it is eaten whole, raw or cooked.

For diners interested in variety, carrots can be baked, cooked, mashed, or used in soups. Carrot croquettes can be made by mashing cooked carrots and adding nutmeg, an egg or two, and some butter. The mixture is then shaped into a carrot form, rolled in bread crumbs, wheat germ flakes or similar dry product, and then chilled for two or three hours. They are then immersed into some pure hot vegetable oil and deep-fried at 380°F until browned. They should then be drained on absorbent paper. By adding a sprig of parsley at the top of each carrot, it will appear to be a freshly plucked carrot direct from the garden. A delightful treat!

A carrot souffle is prepared by mashing two cups of cooked carrots and stirring them into a mixture of three egg yolks, a cup of hot milk and three tablespoons of melted butter. After it has cooled, the three egg whites should be beaten until stiff and then folded into the mixture. It is then all poured into a greased casserole or mold, placed in a pan of hot water, and baked in a moderate oven of 350°F for forty to fifty minutes.

Carrots are often simply placed in the same pan as a pot roast or other meat that is being baked under a cover. The carrots turn brown and go very well with the meat. The carrots are often sprinkled with salt, pepper, or other seasonings.

A highly nourishing soup, with carrots as the main vegetable, is prepared by first heating two tablespoons of vegetable oil in a large soup kettle, browning a large sliced onion in the oil, then adding a tablespoon of whole wheat flour, four cups of beef broth and stir while heating to the boiling point. Boil for two minutes, add a cup of minced celery, one-quarter teaspoon of pepper, four cups of sliced carrots, and allow to simmer for one hour. Serves six.

CASABA MELON

Botanical information: A muskmelon of the family *cucumis malo*.
Nutritive values:

Vitamin A: 30 mg.   Fat: trace
Vitamin B: Thiamine .04 mg.;   Calories: 27
   Riboflavin .03 mg.; Niacin .6 mg.   Carbohydrates: 6.5 gm.
Vitamin C: 13 mg.   Calcium: 14 mg.
Protein: 1.2 gm.   Iron: .4 mg.
                                         Phosphorus: 16 mg.

Reported health benefits: This melon has the same health attributes as the honeydew melon and cantaloupe.
Preparation: The melon can be eaten sliced or it may be cubed and mixed with other fruits and vegetables.

CASHEW NUTS

Botanical information: This nut is the fruit of the tropical American tree *Anacardium occidentale* of the cashew family *Anacardiacae*.

Nutritive values:

Vitamin A: none   Fat: 48.2 gm.
Vitamin B: Thiamine .63 mg.;   Carbohydrates: 27 gm.
   Riboflavin .19 mg.; Niacin 2.1   Calcium: 46 mg.
   mg.   Iron: 5 mg.
Vitamin C: none   Phosphorus: 428 mg.
Protein: 18.5 gm.
Calories: 578

Reported health benefits: The cashew nut and cashew nut butter are good body builders. It is easily digested when eaten raw. Cashews have been reported to be helpful in cases of emaciation, problems with teeth and gums, and when there is a lack of vitality.

Preparation: Cashews are highly nutritious, but when boiled in oil and salted they become somewhat difficult to digest. This food is best combined with acid fruits and nonstarchy vegetables rather than with sweet fruits, proteins or starchy items.

CAULIFLOWER

Botanical information: *Brassica oleracea botrytis* (A cultivated variety of cabbage)

Nutritive values:

Vitamin A: 900 mg.

Vitamin B: Thiamine .11 mg.; Riboflavin .10 mg.; Niacin .6 mg.

Vitamin C: 69 mg.

Protein: 2.4 gm.

Calories: 25

Fat: .2 gm.

Carbohydrates: 4.9 gm.

Calcium: 22 mg.

Iron: 1.1 mg.

Phosphorus: 72 mg.

Reported health benefits: This member of the cabbage family has been found to be a good blood purifier and is indicated in cases of asthma, kidney and bladder disorders, obesity, high blood pressure, gout, bad complexion, biliousness and constipation. Eaten raw, it aids bleeding gums. The leaves should be eaten as greens for rich minerals. Because of the high sulphur content of cauliflower, causing indigestion and poor food assimilation, this vegetable should be used in moderation and not combined with other sulphur-rich foods.

Preparation: Raw cauliflower makes a delicious addition to a combination tossed salad made up of your favorite vegetables. Another salad can be made by taking one medium-sized cauliflower and two raw beets and putting these through a food grinder. Add horseradish and onion juice for extra flavor. Moisten with mayonnaise and serve on romaine lettuce. A nourishing and delicious salad is made by taking one cup cauliflower broken into small pieces and mixing with two cups diced apples, six chopped walnuts, and 1/4 cup finely chopped parsley. Serve on lettuce with mayonaisse or lemon juice dressing.

Many people find it difficult to digest raw cauliflower and prefer to eat it cooked. As with all cooked vegetables, proper preparation is important to insure a minimum loss of vitamins and chemical elements. The cauliflower can be cut into small pieces, placed into a pot with a tight-fitting lid to which very little water has been added, and steamed for eight to ten minutes.

For variety, after the cauliflower has steamed it can be put into a baking dish and cheese sprinkled over it. Bake slowly until cheese is melted and slightly browned.

CELERY, BLEACHED

Botanical information: A biennial apiaceous herb (*Apium grave-olens*). Cultivated mainly for its leafstalks.

Nutritive values:

Vitamin A: none

Vitamin B: Thiamine .05 mg.; Riboflavin .04 mg.; Niacin .4 mg.

Vitamin C: 7 mg.

Protein: 2.4 gm.

Calories: 25

Fat: .2 gm.

Carbohydrates: 4.9 gm.

Calcium: 22 mg.

Iron: 1.1 mg.

Phosphorus: 72 mg.

Potassium: 130 mg.

Reported health benefits: Celery has been recommended for diseases of the kidney (nephritis), arthritis, rheumatism, neuritis, constipation, asthma, high blood pressure, catarrh, pyorrhea, diabetes and dropsy. The celery stalk is usually used, but the leaves are eaten for diabetes and the celery root for dropsy, the condition of accumulation of fluid in a body cavity. Celery is also recommended for conditions of brain overwork (brain-fag) and for acidosis, the condition of depletion of the alkaline reserve or bicarbonate content of the body, celery being an alkaline food. The partaking of celery has been recommended for gall stones, obesity, tuberculosis, and for improvement of the teeth, no doubt due to the presence of calcium. It has also been recommended for cases of anemia, no doubt due to the presence of iron, some proteins and Vitamin B.

Celery is one of the best sources of organic calcium. Nutritionists believe that although calcium is not lost in the cooking process when a food containing calcium is cooked, the calcium is converted into inorganic atoms which are not soluble in water and consequently clog up the system with gall and kidney stones and produce arthritis, coronary distress, and may even cause diabetes and varicose veins by clogging the tiny blood vessels and lymph-carrying passages of the body.

In addition to calcium, celery stalks and juice provide magnesium and sodium. Celery is said to quiet the nerves and to give relief in cases of insomnia. The stalks are considered to be more valuable than the branches.

CHARD

Botanical information: A variety of white beet (*Beta cicla*) cultivated for its large leaves, leafstalks and midribs.

Nutritive values:

Vitamin A: 2,800 I.U. per 100 gm. (The nutritive values are given in this table for leaves and stalks together. Where the leaves alone are used, the Vitamin A value is 8,720 I.U. per 100 gm. There is only a minor difference with regard to other values of leaves alone as compared to the use of leaves and stalks together.)

Vitamin B: Thiamine .06 mg.; Riboflavin .07 mg.; Niacin .4 mg.
Vitamin C: 38 mg.
Protein: 1.4 gm. (2.6 gm. for leaves only)
Calories: 21
Fat: .4 gm.
Carbohydrates: 4.4 gm.
Calcium: 105 mg.
Iron: 2.5 mg.
Phosphorus: 36 mg.

Reported health benefits: Chard has been recommended in cases of anemia, constipation, catarrh, obesity, and poor appetite. Because of chard's high oxalic acid content, this vegetable should be eaten sparingly. Organic oxalic acid (uncooked) is an important element in maintaining the eliminative organs, keeping them in proper tone and stimulating peristaltic action to force out the feces from the body. (When in the cooked or inorganic state, the oxalic acid-rich foods are most destructive of calcium.)

Preparations: While the young leaves can be added as an interesting addition to any salad, as they become more mature the taste becomes rather bitter and the leaves toughen, so it can then be cooked in a number of ways. The basic cooking is like that of spinach: wash in cold water, then place into a saucepan. Do not add water; cover tightly to prevent loss of steam and cook over low heat for ten to fifteen minutes. Drain and serve with salt, pepper and butter. The chard can be served with a cheese sauce by simply browning one tablespoon minced onion and one thin slice garlic in butter, stir in two tablespoons flour and cook until smooth. Add spinach and simmer five minutes; add one cup milk and cook 3 (three) minutes, stirring constantly. Garnish with egg slices.

A delicious ring can be made by melting two tablespoons of butter, blend in two tablespoons of flour, add one-half cup milk and cook until thickened. Add three beaten egg yolks to this mixture. Add one and three-quarters cups cooked chard, salt, pepper, and one-half teaspoon grated onion. Cook for one minute and then fold in stiffly beaten egg whites. Pour into greased ring mold, place in pan of hot water and bake in moderate oven (350 degrees) for about thirty minutes or until firm. Unmold and fill center with creamed fish or vegetables. This will serve six people.

CHERIMOYA

Botanical information: The heart-shaped, scaly, pulpy fruit of a small tree, *anona cherimolia,* grown in Colombia and Peru.

Nutritive values:

Vitamin A: 10 I.U. per 100 gm.
Vitamin B: Thiamine .10 mg.; Riboflavin .11 mg.; Niacin 1.3 mg.
Vitamin C: 9 mg.
Protein: 1.3 gm.
Calories: 94
Fat: .4 gm.
Carbohydrates: 24 gm.
Calcium: 23 mg.
Iron: .5 mg.
Phosphorus: 40 mg.

Reported health benefits: Cherimoya fruit has been found to be beneficial in cases of constipation, halitosis, acidosis, and kidney and bladder inflammation.

Preparation: Cut lengthwise in halves or quarters, depending on the size of the serving you wish to have. Just serve as is; this delectable fruit needs nothing but its own flavor to be complete.

If you want to do something more, scoop out the meat, remove the seeds and use in blender drinks, your favorite sherbet recipe, or with other fruits.

CHERRIES

Botanical information: The cherry is the fruit of the tree or shrub of the genus *Prunus.*

Nutritive values:

Vitamin A: 620 I.U. per 100 gm.　　Fat: .5 gm.
Vitamin B: Thiamine .05 mg.;　　Carbohydrates: 14.8 gm.
　Riboflavin .06 mg.; Niacin .4 mg.　Calcium: 18 mg.
Vitamin C: 8 mg.　　　　　　　　Iron: .4 mg.
Protein: .5 gm.　　　　　　　　Phosphorus: 20 mg.
Calories: 61

Reported health benefits: Cherries are a good "spring" cleaner (the darker cherries being more valuable to the system as they contain a greater quantity of magnesium and iron, and much silicon) and valuable in cases of anemia, poor complexion, bad blood, catarrh, constipation, cramps, obesity, worms, high blood pressure, rheumatism and asthma. They also stimulate the secretion of digestive juices and of the urine and are effective cleansers of the liver and kidneys. Eating large quantities of cherries, from one-half pound and up daily, has been found to bring relief to sufferers of gout, a disease that is characterized by an excess of uric acid in the blood and attacks of arthritis.

Preparation: When being eaten for medicinal purposes it is best to take the cherries uncooked, freshly picked when possible, and very ripe. Also, cherry juice is a very healthful drink, cherry concentrate being available in all health food stores.

A favorite of everyone is cherry pie, especially when homemade and right from the oven. The standard recipe can be made more healthful and tasty by using a wholewheat crust rather than one made with white flour. A good crust can be made by sifting together one and one-half cups wholewheat flour with one-half teaspoon salt. Blend in one-half cup oil and add three tablespoons ice water. Mix thoroughly until it forms a ball of dough. Divide in half and then roll each half one-eighth inch thick. Your filling is made by mixing one and a quarter cups sugar (less if honey is used), two and a half tablespoons flour, one-quarter teaspoon salt, and one quart tart red cherries, washed and pitted. Put cherry mixture into unbaked pastry shell and cover with top crust. Bake in very hot oven (450 degrees) ten minutes; reduce temperature to moderate (350 degrees) and bake twenty-five minutes longer.

To enjoy cherries all year round, they can also be made into a preserve. Heat one cup of sugar with two cups of water and boil five minutes, add fruit and cook until tender. Add one cup of sugar and cook rapidly until thick. Skim and pour into sterile jars. Seal. This will make about one and one-half pints.

A delicious molded salad is made by heating two cups of cherry juice and water, adding one package cherry gelatin and stirring until dissolved. Chill until it begins to thicken and then add two cups cooked cherries, one cup blanched almonds and eight stuffed olives, chopped. Pour into a mold and chill until firm. Unmold and serve in lettuce cups with salad dressing.

Spiced cherries are made by mixing two cups vinegar and eight cups sugar, and boiling for one minute. Skim and then add five pounds cherries and simmer for one and a half hours. Add three tablespoons cinnamon and one and a half tablespoons cloves; mix well. Pour into sterile jars and seal. Makes about eight pints.

CHESTNUT

Botanical information: The nut of the chestnut tree, *castanea*.

Nutritive values:

Vitamin A: none	Fat: 4.1 gm.
Vitamin B: Thiamine .22 mg.;	Calcium: 27 mg.
Riboflavin .22 mg.; Niacin .6 mg.	Iron: 3.8 mg.
Vitamin C: none	Phosphorus: 373 mg.
Protein: 2.9 gm.	
Calories: 377	

Reported health benefits: Chestnuts are good body builders and recommended in cases of emaciation (wasting away of body tissues); also aiding in the care of the teeth and to help cure pyorrhea.

Preparation: Chestnuts should never be eaten raw because of the tannic acid content. They are delicious eaten roasted, hot from the fire. They also make a wonderful addition to dressing for turkey or chicken. The combination of sweet potatoes and chestnuts is a healthful favorite of many people.

Chestnut soup is made by taking two cups of blanched chestnuts and cook in three cups of water until tender; press through sieve and add two cups scalded milk. Cook two tablespoons minced onions in four tablespoons butter until tender, but not brown; blend in two tablespoons flour, one teaspoon salt, one-quarter teaspoon pepper, one-eighth teaspoon celery salt, and a dash of nutmeg. Add milk and chestnut mixture gradually, stirring constantly. Cook five minutes, add one cup cream, heat to boiling, garnish with parsley and serve.

CHICKPEAS

Botanical information: Chickpeas are also referred to as Garbanzos.

Nutritive values:

Vitamin A: Trace

Vitamin B: Thiamine .55 mg.; Riboflavin .17 mg.; Niacin 1.5 mg.

Vitamin C: 2 mg.

Protein: 20.8 gm.

Calories: 359

Fat: 4.7 gm.

Carbohydrates: 60.9 gm.

Calcium: 92 mg.

Iron: 7.1 mg.

Phosphorus: 375 mg.

Reported health benefits: Garbanzos are rich body building food and valuable to those who are underweight. It is a good source of protein for vegetarians; its mild taste and easy digestibility make it a find food for sick persons not able to eat solids.

Preparation: This legume can be substituted in any recipe that calls for any type of dried bean; remember that in order to retain nutritive values and develop full, natural flavor, simmer legumes in water in which they were soaked. Gentle cooking with a minimum of stirring will keep them firm and unbroken. The flavor is enhanced if salt, onions and herbs are added to simmering water. You can prepare enough beans at one time to use for several dishes. Not only are chickpeas delicious in soups and bean-nut loaves, but they are an interesting addition to a tossed salad.

A favorite Middle Eastern recipe for humus, eaten daily, is made by mashing cooked chickpeas and adding lots of garlic lemon juice tahini (a sesame product made from the ground seeds, and olive oil The Arabs have a flat bread with which they scoop up the humus, making a full meal. This is a good hors d'oeuvres recipe, either using flat bread or vegetable sticks for dipping.

COCONUT

Botanical information: The fruit or nut of the coco-palm, having a single seed enclosed in a hard shell with a thick fibrous husk.*Cocos nucifera.*

Nutritive values:

Vitamin A: none

Vitamin B: Thiamine .10 mg.; Riboflavin .01 mg.; Niacin .2 mg.

Fat: 34.7 gm.

Carbohydrates: 14 gm.

Calcium: 21 mg.

Vitamin C: 2 mg.   Iron: 2.0 mg.
Protein: 3.4 gm.   Phosphorus: 98 mg.
Calories: 359

Reported health benefits: In addition to being a good protein food, providing energy and minerals to the body, the meat of the coconut is reported as being valuable for destroying tapeworms acquired by eating infected meat. It is also used generally as a worm destroyer.

Coconuts contain organic iodine and supply the body needs to prevent thyroid gland problems. When the meat is chewed well, the protein content makes it a good body builder and so it is a food recommended for building up the body muscles of thin and emaciated individuals. It is also recommended for constipation and for any build-up of gas in the stomach and intestinal tract and helps cases of dysentery, the condition of inflammation of the large intestine with bloody and loose evacuations.

Coconut milk has been found to help cases of sore throat as well as relieving stomach ulcers.

Coconut oil, prepared by squeezing the juice from the fresh coconut meat, has been found to heal cuts and scratches of the skin as well as heal burns, including sunburns. It has also been recommended as a facial massage and is reported to be good as a wrinkle remover, especially when it is applied after an astringent has been applied to the skin. It is also said to be good for the scalp and hair and makes any hairdressing unnecessary.

Preparation: This fruit has a rich mineral content and is also high in Vitamins A, B, and G. It should be served frequently in any number of interesting ways. It can be sprinkled over all your fruit salads, the flavor of coconut blending nicely with all fruits.

A baked coconut and banana dessert is made by taking six firm bananas, peeling and brushing with lemon juice. Roll the bananas in coconut, place in a greased baking dish, and bake at 375 degrees for fifteen to eighteen minutes.

A favorite and one of the most nourishing desserts is custard. Coconut custard is prepared by taking three eggs and beating slightly, and combining this with one-quarter teaspoon salt and one-third cup sugar. Slowly add three cups scalded milk, stirring constantly, one-half cup shredded coconut and one-half teaspoon vanilla. Pour into custard cups, sprinkle with nutmeg, and place in pan of hot water. This will bake at 350 degrees for thirty to thirty-five minutes, or until a knife inserted in center of custard comes out clean.

A refreshing drink called *"coconut supreme"* is made by liquefying the water from inside a coconut with two cups of crushed pineapple and two cups of pineapple juice, one banana and one cup of freshly grated coconut. Serve one spoonful of grated coconut in each glass.

An unusual recipe from East India is an uncooked coconut soup. Easily made in the blender, take one quart stock, one cup milk, one coconut, one-quarter cup milk powder, one teaspoon flour, juice and rind of one lemon, and one sprig of parsley; blend together until smooth. Chill; when ready to serve, garnish with sprouts of beans, etc.

COLLARDS

Botanical information: A variety of cabbage that does not gather its edible leaves into a head. *Brassica oleracea.*

Nutritive values:

Vitamin A: 6,870 I.U. per 100 gm.   Fat: .6 gm.
Vitamin B: Thiamine .11 mg.;   Carbohydrates: 7.2 gm.
  Riboflavin .27 mg.; Niacin 2 mg.   Calcium: 249 mg.
Vitamin C: 100 mg.   Iron: 1.6 mg.
Protein: 3.9 gm.   Phosphorus: 58 mg.
Calories: 40

Reported health benefits: Because of collards' high alkaline min eral content, this leafy green vegetable has been recommended in cases of anemia, liver trouble, acidosis (excess of acid in the system due to a faulty metabolism), rheumatism, constipation, neuritis, arthritis, obesity, and as an aid in eliminating drug poisoning from the body.

Preparation: Young collard greens can be added to a mixed green salad. To cook collards, wash and drain, and put in boiling salted water; leave uncovered and cook fifteen minutes or until tender. Drain, chop and serve with butter.

Collards with mashed potatoes is prepared by cooking one pound of collard and one pound of potatoes separately. Mash potatoes and mix with minced collards, add butter and beat thoroughly. Fill buttered baking dish and brown in hot oven (450 degrees). Egg yolks may be added before baking.

CORN

Botanical information: In the United States, corn refers to the maize plant or Indian corn. Botanical name of maize is *Zea mays.*

Nutritive values:

Vitamin A: 390 I.U. per 100 gm.

Vitamin B: Thiamine .15 mg.; Riboflavin .12 mg.; Niacin 1.7 mg.

Vitamin C: 12 mg.

Protein: 3.7 gm.

Calories: 92

Fat: 1.2 gm.

Carbohydrates: 20.5 gm.

Calcium: 9 mg.

Iron: .5 mg.

Phosphorus: 120 mg.

Reported health benefits: Corn has been advised in cases of anemia, constipation, emaciation, and as a general building food.

Preparation: The best way to eat corn is uncooked, right off the cob. You will enjoy the delicious taste of the natural sugars and benefit from all the vitamins and minerals. When it is to be cooked, place the stripped corn into boiling water for two to three minutes and then chew thoroughly to insure proper digestion of this starchy food. The corn can also be roasted in an open fire, leaving the corn in its jacket. However you decide to prepare this wonderful vegetable, it is very important that it be as fresh as possible. The older the corn, the greater the depreciation of Vitamins C, A, and B_1, in that order. If the corn is purchased at a market, keep the husks on and put in the refrigerator until ready to use.

If you have a home freezer you will have the opportunity to purchase vegetables in large quantities from local farmers, and by quick freezing, not only will you be able to enjoy your favorite vegetables year round, but you will also benefit from the preserved vitamins and minerals.

A favorite of everyone's is corn chowder. This is easily prepared by taking one-quarter pound of fat salt pork, cut into small pieces and dried out. Add one onion (sliced) and cook until tender. Add three cups diced boiled potatoes, two cups boiling water, one cup cooked corn and four cups hot milk. Season with salt and pepper and heat to boiling. Serve garnished with parsley. This will serve six to eight people.

Corn fritters are made by taking one cup flour, one teaspoon caking powder, three-quarter teaspoon salt, one-quarter teaspoon paprika and sifting together. Add two cups cooked corn and two beaten egg yolks; fold in two stiffly beaten egg whites. Fry in deep fat (365 degrees) until browned. Drain on absorbent paper.

Many people enjoy creamed corn for variety. This is made by combining three cups uncooked corn with one cup cream, one-half teaspoon salt and one-eighth teaspoon pepper. Simmer ten minutes.

This will serve six people. Milk can be used instead of cream; add two tablespoons butter, if desired.

To make Southern Corn Pudding, combine three cups uncooked corn, three eggs (slightly beaten), one teaspoon salt, one-eighth teaspoon pepper, three tablespoons melted fat, three tablespoons sugar, and one and one-eighth cups scalded milk. Pour into greased baking dish and bake in slow oven (325 degrees) thirty to forty minutes or until firm. This recipe serves six to eight persons. You may add one-half cup chopped nuts and two teaspoons grated onion if you like.

CRANBERRY

Botanical information: The bright-scarlet acid berry of two distinct species of *Vaccinium,* the *macrocarpon* and the *oxycoccus.*

Nutritive values:

Vitamin A: 40 I.U. per 100 gm.
Vitamin B: Thiamine .03 mg.;
   Riboflavin .02 mg.; Niacin .1 mg.
Vitamin C: 12 mg.
Protein: .4 gm.
Calories: 48

Fat: .7 gm.
Carbohydrates: 11.3 gm.
Calcium: 14 mg.
Iron: .6 mg.
Phosphorus: 11 mg.

Reported health benefits: Cranberries have been found to be beneficial in cases of skin disorder, both pimples and skin disease; for high blood pressure, constipation, obesity, poor appetite, and fevers. Cranberries are also recommended when there are kidney or liver disturbances. This fruit has a very high acid count, especially tannic and oxalic acids. When overcooked or when there is an addition of sugar to the cranberries, they are exceedingly acid-forming and should be avoided.

Preparation: A fruit salad dressing can be made in the blender by taking two-thirds cup raw cranberries, two tablespoons sweet cider, three tablespoons honey, one tablespoon lemon juice, one-third cup yogurt and three tablespoons oil, and blending until smooth.

Raw cranberry relish is made easily by grinding together two cups cranberries, one-half cup sweet cider, four tablespoons honey, one-quarter teaspoon allspice, pinch of clove. For variation you may add one apple with skin, quartered and cored; one cup fresh diced pineapple; one-half cup diced celery or cucumber; one-half cup chopped raisins; or one-half cup chopped nuts.

This cranberry-apple relish recipe is cooked, so you must be careful not to overcook, and although very tasty, to avoid indigestion do not overeat. Simmer gently one pound cranberries, one cup cider and two apples with skin, sliced, until fruit is soft. Add one cup honey, some lemon rind (grated), and a pinch of ground mace. Simmer for five minutes and cool. This will make two pints that can be served with meat, fowl or fish.

CUCUMBER

Botanical information: Hard-rinded fruit of the cucumber plant *(Cucumis stativus)* cultivated as a vegetable since the days of Moses.

Nutritive values:

Vitamin A: 180 I.U. per 100 gm.

Vitamin B: Thiamine .02 mg.; Riboflavin .04 mg.; Niacin, trace.

Vitamin C: 9 mg.

Protein: .9 gm.

Calories 70

Fat: .2 gm.

Carbohydrates: 17 gm.

Calcium: 32 mg.

Iron: 1.8 mg.

Phosphorus: 27 mg.

Potassium: 80 mg.

Reported health benefits: It has been said that the cucumber is the best natural diuretic known, secreting and promoting the flow of urine. The potassium content of the cucumber makes it highly useful for conditions of both high and low blood pressure. Among other enzymes, the cucumber contains erepsin, the enzyme that helps to digest proteins.

The high silicon and sulphur content of the cucumber is said to promote the growth of hair, especially when the juice of the cucumber is added to the juice of the carrot, lettuce and spinach. A mixture of cucumber juice with carrot juice is said to be very beneficial for rheumatic conditions resulting from excessive uric acid in the body. Cucumber juice is also valuable for helping diseases of the teeth and gums, especially in cases of pyorrhea. The high mineral content of this vegetable also helps to prevent splitting of nails of the fingers or toes.

Preparation: Cucumbers make a good base for a number of salads. To make a cucumber and radish salad, arrange on a plate in this order: six tomatoes, thinly sliced; three cucumbers, sliced; two shredded green peppers; one bunch of radishes, sliced. Top with sour cream dressing and serve.

For a stuffed cucumber salad, take one medium-size cucumber for each serving and slice off the bottom side lengthwise so cucumber will stand straight on salad plate. Cut a wedge-shaped section from the top of each. Mix the cucumber pulp with two tablespoons mayonnaise, one-quarter cup finely chopped celery, and stuff the cucumber shells. Garnish with cream cheese balls and tomato slices. Serve on salad plate with watercress.

A delicious nut and cucumber salad is made simply by placing on a bed of watercress a mixture of one-quarter cup of ground nuts and one small finely chopped cucumber. Mix with a nut dressing and serve.

Yogurt and cucumber soup is made by taking two cucumbers and either grating finely or putting into the blender and puree. Place two cups of yogurt in a large mixing bowl and gradually stir in cucumber puree, one tablespoon tarragon vinegar, lemon juice, one tablespoon olive oil, and one and one-half tablespoons fresh chopped dill. Season with salt and pepper and chill for one hour. When ready to serve, scatter a little dill over each serving.

CURRANT

Botanical information: A small round berry of any species of *Ribes,* a genus of the saxifrage family *(Saxifragaceae)* without prickles and growing in clusters, like grapes.

Nutritive values:

Vitamin A: 120 I.U. per 100 gm.	Fat: .2 gm.
Vitamin B: Thiamine .04 mg.; Riboflavin, none; Niacin, none.	Carbohydrates: 13.6 gm. Calcium: 36 mg.
Vitamin C: 36 mg.	Iron: .9 mg.
Protein: 1.2 gm.	Phosphorus: 33 mg.
Calories: 55	

Reported health benefits: The juice of the currant has an antiseptic effect, and this fruit can be made into one of the most popular liquids for use as a gargle for the throat and as a cough syrup.

Currants have also been recommended as valuable for cases of anemia, constipation, asthma, low blood pressure, tuberculosis, debility, and a weak heart.

Preparation: When cooked with sugar, currants lose much of their medicinal value, and when made into jams and jellies they tend to become acid-forming. As a dried fruit it makes a valuable addition to fruit and vegetable salads, blender drinks, or just eaten by the

handful with almonds or some other kind of nut. Instead of candy, a
nutritional and delicious treat for the children are currant balls. Just
grind the currants, and mix and roll in freshly grated coconut.

DANDELION GREENS

Botanical information: A perennial or biennial milky herb *(Taraxacum taraxacum)* of the aster family, with a large yellow many-
flowered head, solitary on a slender hollow scape or stem.

Nutritive values:

Vitamin A: 13,650 I.U. per 100 gm.   Fat: 2.7 gm.
Vitamin B: Thiamine .19 mg.;   Carbohydrates: 8.8 gm.
  Riboflavin .14 mg.; Niacin .8 mg.   Calcium: 187 mg.
Vitamin C: 36 mg.   Iron: 3.1 mg.
Protein: 2.7 gm.   Phosphorus: 70 mg.
Calories: 44

Reported health benefits: Dandelion greens have been recommended for cleansing of the liver, gallbladder and the spleen. This
plant has also been recommended for anemia, low blood pressure,
poor circulation, emaciation, constipation, eczema, acidosis, and as a
good general tonic and appetizer. One author has stated that
dandelion greens will also help cases involving malignant tumors,
although this has not been recognized by the National Cancer
Institute.

The dandelion greens, made into a tea, have also been found
valuable for treating colds, diabetes, rheumatism, arthritis and kidney
ailments.

Dandelion has also been mentioned for the treatment of syphilis
and gonorrhea.

Preparation: Dandelion greens can be used in salads or prepared
like spinach.

To make dandelion leaf salad in orange and soy dressing, choose
one pound of dandelion leaves that are small and young, wash
carefully and dry. Place in a bowl one-half cup orange juice, one
teaspoon grated orange peel, two tablespoons soy sauce, one teaspoon grated fresh ginger, three tablespoons olive oil, one clove garlic
(mashed), and salt and pepper. Mix these ingredients well. When
ready to serve, pour over the leaves, toss well, and serve at once.

An easy spread to make in the blender is prepared by taking one
cup young dandelion greens, one-half cup cottage cheese, one-quarter

cup nuts, and your favorite dressing, adding enough dressing to make the mixture the right consistency to spread. This will make one and three-quarter cups.

Dandelion greens are objected to because of their sometimes bitter taste. This can be avoided by draining off the first cooking water, then proceeding to cook as planned, adding oil and lemon.

DATE

Botanical information: The fruit of the date palm *(Phoenix dactylifera)*.

Nutritive values:

Vitamin A: 60 I.U. per 100 gm.
Vitamin B: Thiamine .09 mg.; Riboflavin .10 mg.; Niacin 2.2 mg.
Vitamin C: none
Protein: 2.2 gm.
Calories: 284

Fat: .6 gm.
Carbohydrates: 75.4 gm.
Calcium: 72 mg.
Iron: 2.1 mg.
Phosphorus: 60 mg.
Potassium: 1,300 mg.

Reported health benefits: Dates are a highly concentrated and nourishing food, and easily digested as well. They have been found valuable for cases of anemia, low blood pressure, stomach ulcers, piles, colitis, pyorrhea, tuberculosis, sexual impotency, and nervous conditions. They are especially recommended for nursing mothers. Pitted dates, crushed and made into a syrup, have been found beneficial for coughs, sore throat and bronchitis.

Preparation: This fruit is one of the richest in naturally healthful carbohydrates. They are a valuable substitute for candy and not acid-forming. They make an excellent addition to any salad, and can substitute for bread and other carbohydrates at meals.

Rice and date pudding is made by taking one cup cooked brown rice, three cups warmed milk, one-half cup chopped dates, three eggs (well beaten), and three tablespoons honey; mix all ingredients and pour into custard cups. Place cups in pan of hot water and bake in a quick oven until set.

An easy dessert of date pudding can be prepared by taking two cups chopped pitted dates and combining with two cups whipped cream. Add one teaspoon lemon juice and chill thoroughly before serving.

A nourishing drink and perfect mid-afternoon pickup can be made in a liquefier. Take five dates that have been pitted and cut in half, one glass of milk, one teaspoon powdered coconut and one teaspoon nuts. Liquefy and serve.

Any number of fruit spread combinations can be made; for instance, date nut spread is made in the blender by taking one cup pitted dates, one-half cup nuts, one-quarter cup yogurt, and one-half cup powdered milk. Blend and then keep refrigerated until ready to use. For a spiced spread, add one-half teaspoon ground cinnamon.

Date orange spread is made by placing two cups pitted dates, one teaspoon powdered fruit ring, juice of one orange and one-quarter cup wheat germ in a blender and mixing until smooth. If too thin to spread, add more wheat germ.

To your favorite loaf cake, bread, or cooked cereal, dates can be added for extra nutrition and wonderful taste treat.

DULSE

Botanical information: Plant of the class *Algae* living in the sea, of type *Laurencia pinnatifida.*

Nutritive values:

Vitamin A: none

Vitamin B: none

Vitamin C: none

Protein: 25.3 gm.

Calories: none

Fat: 3.2 gm.

Calcium: 296 mg.

Iron: 150.0 mg.

Phosphorus: 240 mg.

Reported health benefits: Dulse has the same medicinal properties as kelp. Very high in mineral content, it is an especially good source of iodine, potassium and sodium.

Preparation: Dulse may be purchased in powder form, combined with kelp; in tablets; or dried in leaf form. It may be sprinkled on all foods, replacing salt. The dried leaves may be soaked in water for several minutes and then chopped and added to salad.

EGGPLANT

Botanical information: An herb of the nightshade family *(Solanum melongena)* with large egg-shaped edible fruit (berries), commonly purple.

Nutritive values:

Vitamin A: 30 I.U. per 100 gm.

Vitamin B: Thiamine .04 mg.; Riboflavin .05 mg.; Niacin .65 mg.

Vitamin C: 5 mg.

Protein: 1.1 gm.

Calories: 24

Fat: .2 gm.

Carbohydrates: 5.5

Calcium: 15 mg.

Iron: .4 mg.

Phosphorus: 37 mg.

Potassium: 390 mg.

Reported health benefits: Eggplant has been found valuable for cases of constipation, colitis, stomach ulcers and various nervous conditions.

Preparation: Eggplant should not be fried. They are much more easily digested when baked plain or in a casserole, mixed with cheese. A simple preparation of eggplant to serve with lamb or veal is made by slicing small, unpeeled eggplant about one-quarter inch thick, and brushing with oil. Place on sheet and let bake about ten minutes. Turn and sprinkle top of slices with parsley and place a cube of mozzarella cheese in the center. Let bake another ten minutes, or you can bake both sides until done, add the cheese and parsley, and slip under the broiler until the cheese melts.

A number of main-course casseroles can be made with eggplant in combination with other vegetables and cheeses. A basic casserole recipe is prepared by taking one and one-half pounds diced eggplant and three medium onions that have been chopped; cover with boiling water and cook about twenty minutes. Drain and add to this two tablespoons butter, two beaten egg yolks, one-half cup grated Parmesan cheese, one teaspoon salt, and one cup of dry bread crumbs. Pour into a greased baking dish and cook for thirty minutes in a moderate oven (350 degrees). To this recipe you may add squash, okra, or tomatoes for variety. For an Italian flavor, oregano and basil may be added to the mixture and a few minutes before the casserole is through baking, slices of mozzarella cheese can be placed on top and the dish placed back in the oven until the cheese melts.

An excellent accompaniment to lamb dishes or any hearty meat dish is marinated eggplant with olives and hard-boiled eggs. Choose one small, tender eggplant and dice. Put this in two tablespoons cider vinegar and marinate for two hours. Combine in a dish the eggplant, one onion (finely chopped), chopped fresh basil and parsley, and one cup pitted black olives. Season the eggplant with salt and pepper and turn in two tablespoons of olive oil. When ready to serve, garnish with two hard-boiled eggs that have been sliced.

ELDERBERRY

Botanical information: Purple-black drupaceous fruit of the common elder (genus *Sambucus*).

Nutritive values:

Vitamin A: 600 I.U. per 100 gm.
Vitamin B: Thiamine .07 mg.;
   Riboflavin .06 mg.; Niacin .5 mg.
Vitamin C: 36 mg.
Protein: 2.6 gm.
Calories: 72

Fat: .5 gm.
Carbohydrates: 16.4 gm.
Calcium: 38 mg.
Iron: 1.6 mg.
Phosphorus: 28 mg.

Reported health benefits: Elderberries are recommended in cases of bronchitis, sore throats, coughs, asthma, colds, catarrh, and constipation. They also induce perspiration.

Preparation: The most common use of elderberries is in the making of wine and jelly.

ENDIVES

Botanical information: An herb *(Cichorium endivia).* The leaves are used as a salad. Another variety is endive escarole, a variety of chicory *(Cichorium intybus).*

Nutritive values:

√itamin A: 3,000 I.U. per 100 gm.
Vitamin B: Thiamine .06 mg.
Vitamin C: 11 mg.
Protein: 1.6 gm.
Calories: 20

Fat: .2 gm.
Carbohydrates: 4 gm.
Calcium: 79 mg.
Iron: 1.7 mg.
Phosphorus: 56 mg.
Potassium: 28 mg.

Reported health benefits: This vegetable has been found useful in cases of asthma, tuberculosis, skin infections, gout, diabetes, constipation, obesity, rheumatism, anemia, high blood pressure, catarrh (secretions from mucous membranes), liver ailments, arthritis, neuritis, acidosis, and stomach gas or biliousness.

Preparation: Likeother members of the chicory family, endive is a valuable addition to a salad. Its bitter flavor stimulates the secretion of saliva and of bile; its rich mineral content, especially potassium, sodium, calcium, and phosphorous, makes it very nourishing to the optic system.

FIG 99

Alone, endive can be served with a roquefort dressing or an orange and soy dressing. The leaves of endive should never be washed, as this tends to make them bitter. Cut off the bottom part and discard the brown outer leaves. Then take the leaves off separately and wipe away any dirt with a paper towel. Put leaves in a bowl and pour the dressing over and serve immediately. Endive goes brown if exposed to the air.

For hors d'oeuvres, stuff the leaves of endive with roquefort cheese. Take two medium-size heads of endive and pull the leaves off. Wipe the leaves and squeeze a little lemon juice over them. Mix one-half cup roquefort cheese with one-quarter cup heavy cream and stuff the leaves with the mixture, sprinkling the whole with black pepper and garnishing with black olives and halved baby tomatoes.

For those who do not care for the strong flavor of roquefort cheese, the endive could be stuffed with cottage cheese and served in a like manner as above with French dressing.

FIG

Botanical information: The common fig *Ficus carica)* is of Oriental origin, being a small tree with large leaves and cultivated from very ancient times.

Nutritive values:

Vitamin A: 80 I.U. per 100 gm.	Fat: .4 gm.
Vitamin B: Thiamine .06 mg.;	Carbohydrates: 19.6 gm.
.Riboflavin .05 mg.; Niacin .5 mg.	Calcium: 54 mg.
Vitamin C: 2 mg.	Iron .6 mg.
Protein: 1.4 gm.	Phosphorus: 32 mg.
Calories: 79	

Reported health benefits: Figs have been found beneficial for constipation, low blood pressure, anemia, colitis, emaciation, asthma, tuberculosis, pleurisy, catarrh, gout, rheumatism, and skin diseases. It is also said to be helpful in cases of Ryanaud's disease, where there is suspended animation of the arms and legs, apparently resulting from poor circulation. Fig juice from soaked figs is reported as an excellent laxative and also beneficial for sore throats, coughs, and ulcers in the digestive system.

By splitting open a fig and soaking it for several minutes in warm water, the fig forms an excellent poultice for an external inflamed boil or othr abscess. It also may be applied with generally good results to an abscess of the gums of the teeth.

Preparation: When fresh figs are in season they should be eaten abundantly, especially by children, for their high mineral content (two or four times higher than that of most fresh foods). Because figs are highly perishable they are not shipped to any great extent, but are usually prepared as jams, canned, or dried. The drying of this fruit does not inhibit its nutritional value; in fact, fruits that are sun-dried are found to be nutritionally richer.

Figs with honey is a superb dessert, delicious and easy to prepare during the summer when fresh figs are available. Take sixteen ripe green figs and cut them in quarters. Put three-quarter cup clear honey in a bowl and pour one-half cup boiling water over it. Stir well and add figs, turning them in the mixture. Refrigerate overnight, or at least for an hour, and serve with heavy cream. For another fresh fig dessert (or canned figs can be used, but it won't be as tasty) take about twelve figs, prick holes all over the fruit, and cover them with kirsch (or brandy). Just before serving, set the liqueur on fire so that it loses its harsh edge and impregnates the figs. This dramatic dessert will serve four persons.

To make individual steamed fig puddings, take enough figs that when put through a food chopper they will amount to three-quarters of a cup. Cream three-quarters cup shortening and one cup sugar together until fluffy. Add two beaten eggs and mix; add figs, blending well. Sift two cups flour, one-half teaspoon salt, one teaspoon baking soda, one teaspoon mace, and one teaspoon cinnamon together. Add alternately with one-half cup sour milk in small amounts, mixing well after each addition. Stir in one teaspoon vanilla and pour into greased custard cups, filling slightly over one-half full. Cover and steam for forty-five minutes. This should be served hot with lemon, vanilla or marshmallow sauce.

A wonderful confection for the children is made by taking the desired number of white figs, cut off about three-quarters of the stem end, and open to stuff. Put equal parts fresh coconut and sesame seed through a food chopper. Add a little nuts and stuff each fig fully. Garnish each fig with a pine nut.

FILBERTS

Botanical information: Filbert is the edible nut of the European or Oriental Hazel *(corylus acellana* or *corylus pontica).*

Nutritive values:

Vitamin A: none   Fat: 62.4 gm.

Vitamin B: Thiamine .46 mg.; Carbohydrates: 16.7 gm.
  Riboflavin, none; Niacin .9 mg. Calcium: 209 mg.
Vitamin C: trace Iron: 3.4 mg.
Proteins: 12.6 gm Phosphorus: 337 mg.
Calories: 634

Reported health benefits: Filberts are a rich food for those with good digestion. Whereas most nuts have an alkaline reaction on the system, filberts, along with peanuts and walnuts, are acid-forming, and should be eaten in moderation. They are very good for the teeth and gums, and aid in normalizing the metabolism and building a strong body.

Preparation: Eat filberts right from the shell as a snack, or substitute them for any other nut called for in nut and vegetable entrees. When making a loaf from nuts, always use fresh, raw, unoiled and unsalted nuts. Grind small quantities as needed. Since nuts are very perishable, they should be either left in their shells or refrigerated until used.

GARLIC

Botanical information: A hardy bulbous perennial *(Allium sativum)* of the lily family. The bulb is composed of ten to twelve small cloves.

Nutritive values:

Vitamin A: Trace. Fat: .2 gm.
Vitamin B: Thiamine .25 mg.; Carbohydrates: 30.8 gm.
  Riboflavin .08 mg.; Niacin .5 mg. Calcium: 29 mg.
Vitamin C: 15 mg. Iron: 1.5 mg.
Protein: 6.2 gm. Phosphorus: 202 mg.
Calories: 137 Potassium: 29 mg.

Reported health benefits: Garlic is one of the most beneficial foods for the digestive system and has a good effect on the lymph, aiding in the elimination of noxious waste matter in the body. It is also a useful cleanser of the blood, therefore helpful in conditions of high blood pressure. It tends to stimulate peristaltic action and the secretion of the digestive juices. Garlic has been found useful in cases of colds, asthma, chronic catarrh, bronchitis, fevers, gas, hardening of the arteries, thyroid hypo-function, sinusitis, and promotes the expectoration of phlegm and mucus.

Eat it raw when possible—parsley, mint or orange peelings, when chewed after the meal, help to eliminate the odor.

Preparation: The subtle suggestion of garlic improves almost every recipe, enhancing the natural flavors of meats and vegetables, so that little or no additional seasoning is required.

Chicken can be rubbed both inside and out with crushed garlic and then left at room temperature for half an hour so that the garlic permeates the meat; roasts can also be rubbed with the crushed garlic, making a good salt substitute.

In salad preparation, first rub your wooden bowl with garlic; for additional flavor, add sliced cloves of garlic to the salad dressing and let sit for several hours before putting on salad, removing the garlic first.

Always use fresh garlic in cooking. The powdered garlic not only is less flavorful, but also is missing the valuable nutrients that fresh cloves of garlic contain.

GOOSEBERRY

Botanical information: The fruit of any spiny shrub of the genus *Grossularia.*

Nutritive values:

Vitamin A: 290 I.U. per 100 gm.	Fat: .2 gm.
Vitamin B: none	Carbohydrates: 9.7 gm.
Vitamin C: 33 mg.	Calcium: 22 mg.
Protein: .8 gm.	Iron: .5 mg.
Calories: 39	Phosphorus: 28 mg.

Reported health benefits: Gooseberries have been recommended for constipation, liver ailments, gallbladder congestion, obesity, poor complexion, catarrh, neuritis, arthritis, nephritis (inflammation of the kidneys), and dyspepsia (indigestion usually due to excess acid).

Preparation: To make gooseberry jam, take one pound berries, clean, remove stems, and crush slightly for juicing action. Cook until soft, add one pound sugar, heat slowly until sugar is dissolved, then boil rapidly until juice gives test for jelly. Pour into sterile glasses and seal. Makes about two (six ounce) glasses. Testing for jelly is done by taking a little cooked juice on a spoon, cool slightly and pour slowly back into kettle from the edge of the spoon. If the jelly is not cooked sufficiently the juice will fall in two parallel drops. When the jelly is cooked sufficiently the drops run together and fall from the spoon in a flake or sheet, leaving the edge of the spoon clean.

A wonderful treat in the summer is a fresh berry pie, especially if you worked hard all day collecting the berries! To make a gooseberry pie, combine three cups gooseberries with one cup sugar and one-half cup water; cook until the berries are tender. Sift together one-half cup sugar, two tablespoons flour, one-quarter teaspoon salt, one teaspoon cinnamon, one-half teaspoon cloves, and one-eighth teaspoon nutmeg. Stir the sifted ingredients into the cooked mixture and cool. Pour the filling into your favorite pastry crust and dot with butter. Cover with top crust and bake in a very hot oven (450 degrees) for ten minutes; reduce temperature to moderate (350 degrees) and bake twenty-five minutes longer. This will make one nine-inch pie.

An unusual spicy relish to warm up the cold winter months is made simply by taking five pounds of ripe gooseberries which have been washed and picked over; combine with four pounds of brown sugar, two cups vinegar, two tablespoons cloves, three teaspoons cinnamon and three teaspoons allspice. Cook slowly until mixture becomes rather thick; pour into sterile glasses and seal. This recipe will make about five pints.

GRANADILLA FRUIT

Botanical information: Granadilla, also known as passion fruit, is the fruit of a small tree, *passiflora.*

Nutritive values:

Vitamin A: 700 I.U. per 100 gr.   Fat: .7 gm.
Vitamin B: Thiamine, trace; Ribo-   Carbohydrates: 21.2 gm.
   flavin .13 mg.; Niacin 1.5 mg.   Calcium: 13 mg.
Vitamin C: 30 mg.   Iron: 1.6 mg.
Protein: 2.2 gm.   Phosphorus: 64 mg.
Calories: 90

Reported health benefits: This delicious fruit is reported to be beneficial in cases of obesity, tumors, and sluggish liver.

Preparation: This fruit should be eaten very ripe when it is available. It can be added to fruit salads or blender drinks.

GRAPE

Botanical information: The fruit of the grapevine of any one of the many species of the genus *Vitis,* cultivated for eating and for making wine and raisins.

Nutritive values:

Vitamin A: 80 I.U. per 100 gm.   Fat: 1.4 gm.
Vitamin B: Thiamine .06 mg.;   Carbohydrates: 14.9 gm.
   Riboflavin .04 mg.; Niacin .2 mg.   Calcium: 17 gm.
Vitamin C: 4 mg.   Iron: .6 mg.
Protein: 1.4 gm.   Phosphorus: 21 mg.
Calories: 70

Reported health benefits: Grapes are called "the queen of fruits" because of their great internal body cleansing properties. A good blood and body builder, it is a source of quick energy. Grape juice is easily assimilated and called the "nectar of the gods." It is indicated in cases of constipation, gout and rheumatism, skin and liver disorders. This alkaline fruit helps greatly to decrease the acidity of the uric acid and lends itself further in aiding the elimination of the acid from the system, thus benefiting the kidneys greatly.

Preparation: Grapes are often taken as the entire meal, lending to their cleansing properties. They may also be combined with other fruits in a salad or made into juice, jam or jelly.

GRAPEFRUIT

Botanical information: A large, pale yellow citrus fruit, *Citrus decumana.*

Nutritive values:

Vitamin A: Trace   Fat: .2 gm.
Vitamin B: Thiamine .04 mg.;   Carbohydrates: 10.1 gm.
   Riboflavin .02 mg.; Niacin .2 mg.   Calcium: 22 mg.
Vitamin C: 40 mg.   Iron: .2 mg.
Protein: .5 gm.   Phosphorus: 14 mg.
Calories: 40

Reported health benefits: Grapefruit has been found to be one of the most valuable fruits as an aid in the removal or dissolving of inorganic calcium which may have formed in the cartilage of the joints, as in arthritis, as a result of an excessive consumption of devitalized white flour products. Fresh grapefruit contains organic salicylic acid, which aids in dissolving such inorganic calcium in the body. The rinds of the grapefruit should be grated, cut, and dried, and saved for use during the winter as a "cold breaker" made by putting a level teaspoonful of the grated rind in a cup of hot water and steeping, either alone or with equal portions of sage, boneset and mint. This should be taken every hour until the desired results are obtained.

Grapefruit is a natural antiseptic for wounds when used externally, and indicated in cases of obesity, sluggish liver, gall stones, catarrh, fevers, pneumonia, poor digestion, poor complexion, and valuable as a drug-poison eliminator.

Preparation: Grapefruits are best eaten uncooked, either alone or added to a fruit salad. They also may be juiced and drunk alone, or combined with orange or pineapple juice.

GUAVA

Botanical information: The fruit of a tropical American tree, *Psidium guayaba,* family *Myrtaceae.* The fruit resembles the apple and the pear, and is yellow outside and red inside. The pulp is made into guava jelly.

Nutritive values:

Vitamin A: 250 I.U. per 100 gm.
Vitamin B: Thiamine .07 mg.; Riboflavin .04 mg.; Niacin 1.2 mg.
Vitamin C: 302 mg.
Protein: 1.0 gm.
Calories 70

Fat: .6 gm.
Carbohydrates: 17.1 gm.
Calcium: 30 mg.
Iron: .7 mg.
Phosphorus: 29 mg.

Reported health benefits: Indicated in cases of diarrhea, prolonged menstruation, high blood pressure, poor circulation, acidosis, asthma, catarrh, and obesity.

Preparation: Guava can be eaten as a delicious fruit or made into jelly. An easy to make Latin American dessert can be made by taking the guava shells, allowing two to three per person, and serve on a plate with a good portion of cream cheese in the center of each shell. The very sweet taste of the guava contrasts well with the cream cheese, making this a wonderful treat when this exotic fruit is available.

HAW (SCARLET)

Botanical information: Fruit of the hawthorn scrub, *crataegus coccinea,* grown in southern Canada and in the eastern part of the United States.

Nutritive values:

Protein: 2.0 gm. per 100 gm.   Fat: .7 gm
Calories: 87   Carbohydrates: 20.8 gm.

Reported health benefits: Haws are a cleansing fruit and are excellent for cleansing the intestines in cases of constipation, obesity, acidosis, excessive gas, dyspepsia, and high blood pressure.

Preparation: Haws may be eaten raw or made into a salad with other fruits and vegetables.

HICKORY

Botanical information: The hickory nut is the edible seed of any of several North American trees of the genus *Carya.*

Nutritive values:

Protein: 12.6 gm.   Calcium: trace
Calories: 673   Iron: 2.4 mg.
Fat: 62.4 gm.   Phosphorus: 360 mg.
Carbohydrates: 12.8 gm.

Reported health benefits: The hickory nut is one of the richest in nutrients and is a good general body builder, recommended in cases of low vitality, low blood pressure, emaciation and poor teeth.

Preparation: Like all nuts, it is best to eat hickory nuts raw and unsalted, as the roasting process heats the fat in the nut and renders it toxic. They may be eaten right out of the shell as a snack or added to any recipe calling for the addition of nut meat.

HONEYDEW MELON

Botanical information: A muskmelon of the family *cucumis malo.*

Nutritive values:

Vitamin A: 40 mg.   Fat: trace
Vitamin B: Thiamine .04; Ribo-   Carbohydrates: 6.5 gm.
    flavin .03 mg.; Niacin .6 mg.   Calcium: 14 mg.
Vitamin C: 23 mg.   Iron: .4 mg.
Protein: .8 gm.   Phosphorus: 16 mg.
Calories: 27

Reported health benefits: Muskmelons are especially good for kidney conditions because of their diuretic action. They are reported to aid in cases of obesity, rheumatism, and poor complexion.

Preparation: It is recommended that melons be eaten alone and without the addition of salt or sugar. They have a small proportion of cellulose fiber; this makes them easily digestable if no other food interferes with the digestive process.

HORSERADISH

Botanical information: Root of the plant *Roripa armoracia.*

Nutritive values:

Vitamin A: none

Vitamin B: Thiamine .07 mg.; Riboflavin, none; Niacin, none.

Vitamin C: 81 mg.

Protein: 3.1 gm.

Calories: 87

Fat: .3 gm.

Carbohydrates: 19.7 gm.

Calcium: 140 mg.

Iron: 1.4 mg.

Phosphorus: 6.4 mg.

Reported health benefits: Horseradish is one of the most valuable concentrated foods; it is an excellent solvent of excessive mucus in the system, especially in the nasal and sinus cavities. It is recommended for colds, coughs and asthma.

This wonderful vegetable also stimulates appetite as it aids in the secretion of digestive juices. If taken in excess it may be irritating to the kidneys and bladder, so it is advisable to not take more than one-quarter teaspoon at a time. The best preparation of horseradish is to grate it very fine and combine with equal amounts of lemon juice, taking one-quarter teaspoon four times daily.

Preparation: Prepared horseradish may be purchased at all grocery stores; however, to obtain full nutritional benefits, it is advisable to obtain a fresh horseradish root and prepare it yourself as above. It may be combined with butter for sandwiches, used in sauces for meat and fish, or used with other ingredients as a salad dressing.

JACKFRUIT

Botanical information: Fruit of the cultured tree *(artocarpus integridfolia)* of the breadfruit family of Southeast Asia.

Nutritive values:

Vitamin A: none

Vitamin B: Thiamine .03 mg.;
   Riboflavin, none; Niacin .4 mg.

Vitamin C: 8 mg.

Protein: 1.3 gm.

Calories: 98

Fat: .3 gm.

Carbohydrates: 25.4 gm.

Reported health benefits: Jackfruit is an excellent energy food with only a small amount of fat. It is recommended in conditions where there is tension, nervousness, high blood pressure, obesity and constipation.

Preparation: It may be eaten raw or sliced into a salad with other fruits and vegetables.

JERUSALEM ARTICHOKE

Botanical information: The edible tuber of the *helianthus tuberosus* plant.

Nutritive values:

Vitamin A: 20 I.U. per 100 gm.

Vitamin B: Thiamine .20 mg.;
   Riboflavin .06 mg.; Niacin 1.3
   mg.

Vitamin C: 4 mg.

Proteins: 2.3 gm.

Calories: 75

Fat: .1 gm.

Carbohydrates: 16.7 gm.

Calcium: 14 mg.

Iron: 3.4 mg.

Phosphorus: 78 mg.

Reported health benefits: This tuber is recommended in cases of constipation, gas and biliousness. It also has been found beneficial when there is catarrh present in the system. It makes a good potato substitute for diabetics and others who cannot eat potatoes.

Preparation: The Jerusalem artichoke is not related to the globe artichoke as many people believe. It is actually the root of a sunflower plant known as the "Sunflower Artichoke." The tubers are the section eaten, with a nutlike flavor. It may be baked, boiled or used raw. It is also used for making macaroni-style noodles and similar products. It is considered starchless, storing its carbohydrates in the form of inulin, which makes this vegetable valuable for diabetics and those who must limit their starch intake.

To prepare, wash and scrape one and one-half pounds of artichokes and cook in boiling water until tender. After fifteen minutes, test them with a toothpick and drain. Heat two tablespoons oil, add one teaspoon cider vinegar and parsley, pour over sliced artichokes and serve.

To prepare a Jerusalem artichoke souffle, combine two cups hot riced artichokes with one-half cup hot sauce made with milk, butter and flour, and beat thoroughly. Add two beaten egg yolks, one-half teaspoon salt, and one-eighth teaspoon pepper, and beat again. Fold in two stiffly beaten egg whites, pour into greased baking dish, and sprinkle with one tablespoon grated cheese. Bake in moderate oven (350 degrees) about twenty-five minutes.

JUJUBE

Botanical information: Edible fruit of Old World spiny scrubs of genus *Zizyphis,* of the Buckthorn family. Red berries.

Nutritive values:

Vitamin A: 40 I.U. per 100 gm.
Vitamin B: Thiamine .02 mg.;
Riboflavin .04 mg.; Niacin .9 mg.
Vitamin C: 69 mg.
Protein: 1.2 gm.
Calories: 105

Fat: .2 gm.
Carbohydrates: 27.6 gm.
Calcium: 29 mg.
Iron: .5 mg.
Phosphorus: 37 mg.

Reported health benefits: A variety of minerals and vitamins, a fair amount of carbohydrates, and a fairly high caloric value make this an excellent food for obesity, high blood pressure and body building. The high phosphorus content makes this a good food for the nerves and brain. Phosphorus also stimulates growth of bone and hair.

Preparation: The berries may be eaten raw or blended into a delicious fruit drink. They may also be mixed with other fruits and vegetables and made into a salad.

KALE

Botanical information: A variety of headless cabbage, yielding curled and wrinkled leaves. *Brassica oleracea.*

Nutritive values:

Vitamin A: 7,540 I.U. per 100 gm.
Vitamin B: Thiamine .10 mg.;

Fat: .6 gm.
Carbohydrates: 7.2 gm.

Riboflavin .26 mg.; Niacin 2 mg.   Calcium: 225 mg.
Vitamin C: 115 mg.   Iron: 2.2 mg.
Protein: 3.9 gm.   Phosphorus: 62 mg.
Calories: 40

Reported health benefits: This leafy green vegetable has been found to be helpful in cases of constipation, obesity, acidosis, general emaciation, poor teeth, pyorrhea, arthritis, gout, rheumatism, skin diseases, and bladder disorders.

Preparation: When young, this vitamin-rich green is a valuable addition to a raw salad because of its internal body-cleansing properties. It has a tendency to generate gas, so care should be taken not to overindulge in eating this vegetable.

To cook kale, place two pounds of kale, which has been washed and heavy stems removed, in a saucepan. Add enough boiling water to cover kale and cook uncovered twenty-five to thirty-five minutes, or until tender. Drain. To serve, add salt, pepper and butter. This will yield about three and one-half cups.

For scalloped kale, cook as above and combine with three hard-boiled eggs (chopped) and one cup sauce made with milk, butter and flour. Arrange in alternate layers with one cup grated cheese and bake at 400 degrees for fifteen minutes. This will serve six people.

An interesting and tasty combination is kale with sour cream. Place four cups of cooked kale in saucepan; add one tablespoon butter, one teaspoon sugar, one teaspoon salt, one-eighth teaspoon pepper and one teaspoon lemon juice, and heat thoroughly. Reduce heat and stir in sour cream (one cup) gradually.

KELP

Botanical information: A sea vegetable of the *Laminariaceae* type.

Nutritive values:

Vitamin A: 2 I.U. per 100 gm.
Vitamin B: Thiamine, none; Ribo-   Carbohydrates: 40.2 gm.
flavin .33 mg.; Niacin 5.7 mg.   Calcium: 1093 mg.
Protein: 7.5 gm.   Iron: 100 mg.
Fat: 1.1 gm.   Phosphorus: 240 mg.
                                    Also other ocean minerals,
                                    such as iodine, etc.

Reported health benefits: Kelp, either fresh or powdered, is the richest source of organic iodine. It helps correct mineral deficiencies and is a good protective food, valuable in overcoming poor digestion, preventing and overcoming goiter, and rebuilding and maintaining the proper function of all the glands. Kelp has been reported to be an aid in brain development; it offsets deficiencies of an inferior diet; it is beneficial for those suffering from impotency, anemia and emaciation.

Preparation: Kelp may be purchased at all health food stores in powdered form, either alone or combined with dulse and other seasonings. It is an excellent salt substitute and should be kept on the table. It may be sprinkled on salads, vegetables and other foods, adding new flavor and valuable nutrients to the meal.

KOHLRABI

Botanical information: This is a member of the *caulis rapa* family.

Nutritive values:

Vitamin A: 20 I.U. per 100 gm.   Fat: .1 gm.
Vitamin B: Thiamine .06 mg.;   Carbohydrates: 6.6 gm.
   Riboflavin .04 mg.; Niacin .3 mg.   Calcium: 41 mg.
Vitamin C: 66 mg.   Iron: .5 mg.
Protein: 2.0 gm.   Phosphorus: 51 mg.
Calories: 29

Reported health benefits: Kohlrabi is an excellent blood cleanser and is recommended for those with toxemia and resulting poor complexions. It is also reported to be valuable for gums and teeth, for bone development, and for healthy nails. When there is kidney or bladder irritation, kohlrabi has been found to be very beneficial, especially when eaten raw.

Preparation: Kohlrabi is very delicious eaten raw, either by itself or added to a salad.

To cook kohlrabi, pare and cut into cubes or slices two pounds of the vegetable and let stand in water which has two tablespoons of vinegar added to it for an hour. Rinse, place in a saucepan, cover with boiling water, and add one-half teaspoon salt. Cook uncovered for twenty to thirty-five minutes. Drain. Serve seasoned with salt, pepper, and butter, or a hollandaise sauce.

KUMQUAT

Botanical information: Fruit from the *citrus japonica* tree.

Nutritive values:

Vitamin A: 600 mg.
Vitamin B: Thiamine .08 mg.;
  Riboflavin .10.
Vitamin C: 36 mg.
Protein: .9 gm.
Calories: 65

Fat: 1 gm.
Carbohydrates: 17.1 gm.
Calcium: 63 mg.
Iron: .4 mg.
Phosphorus: 23 mg.

Reported health benefits: This member of the orange family has been found to be helpful in cases of obesity, high blood pressure, catarrh, fevers, and pneumonia.

Preparation: This delicious and nourishing fruit should be eaten very ripe, and just as it comes off the tree.

LEEKS

Botanical information: Culinary herb, closely related to the onion, the common garden variety of the *allium porrum* family.

Nutritive values:

Vitamin A: 40 I.U. per 100 gm.
Vitamin B: Thiamine .11 mg.;
  Riboflavin .06 mg.; Niacin .5 mg.
Protein: 2.2 gm.
Calories: 52

Fat: .3 gm.
Carbohydrates: 11.2 gm.
Calcium: 52 mg.
Iron: 1.1 mg.
Phosphorus: 50 mg.

Reported health benefits: The leek is a valuable addition to the diet; having many of the same medicinal properties of garlic, it may be taken by those who find garlic too irritating to the system. It is a good general stimulant, helpful in cases of bronchitis, influenza, insomnia, and low blood pressure.

Preparation: Leeks serve as a green replacement for chives, scallions, onions and garlic tops. It should be served uncooked and should be chewed well.

LEMON

Botanical information: The fruit of the tropical or subtropical tree *Citrus medica limonum,* of the family *Rutaceae.* The rind contains oil of lemon. The juice has citric acid.

Nutritive values:

Vitamin B: Thiamine .04 mg.; Riboflavin, trace; Niacin .1 mg.	Fat: .6 gm.
	Carbohydrates: 8.7 gm.
Vitamin C: 50 mg.	Calcium: 40 mg.
Protein: .9 gm.	Iron: .6 mg.
Calories: 32	Phosphorus: 22 mg.

Reported health benefits: As a natural antiseptic, the juice of the lemon will destroy harmful bacteria found in cuts and other areas of infection. One-half lemon in a quart of warm water may be used as a vaginal douche for general cleansing purposes; however, if the mucous membrane is inflamed, this procedure should be avoided because of the painful discomfort that may result. For skin problems, the juice of the lemon should be applied directly to the skin and allowed to dry, especially for acne, eczema and erysipelas, the skin disease caused by a form of bacteria.

Heating a lemon in an oven and slicing it into two parts, one large and one small, and placing the open end of the small part to a boil or carbuncle (gangrenous tumor) and binding it into position, should result in destruction of bacteria. After about an hour or when the boil breaks, the dressing and pus should be removed and the part cleaned with boiled warm water diluted with lemon juice.

In applying lemon juice directly to blackheads, the dark-colored secretions that clog skin ducts, the juice should be rubbed over the blackheads nightly and allowed to dry without being wiped off. This technique is also applicable to ordinary open sores of the body. It will also help in removal of tan spots on the body, such as freckles, serving as a bleach.

Lemon juice has been recommended for wrinkles, the juice being applied directly to the wrinkle and allowed to dry. After being on the skin for several hours, it is then removed and coconut or olive oil is applied.

Another use for lemon juice is for the prevention of pyorrhea by using it as a dentrifice. It will also remove stains from the teeth. It may be applied by using a knife or scissors to cut the rind into slices and then applying the inside of the rind to the teeth and gums.

Dandruff may be treated by applying lemon juice to the scalp, followed by a shampoo. Again, after the shampoo and wash, take the juice of one lemon and mix it with a glass of water; the solution is excellent for removing soap from the hair and scalp. It also gives a shine to the hair and refreshes the scalp.

Lemon juice has been found to give relief to sore and reddened hands. After massaging with the juice, the juice is washed off and olive oil, coconut oil or vaseline is applied.

Lemon juice is also valuable for relieving the itch of insect bites, as well as the irritation caused by poison oak or ivy.

Equal parts of lemon juice with honey or glycerine, taken every two hours, a tablespoonful at a time, will usually relieve coughs. A sore throat can often be relieved by first drinking some of the lemon juice·(tablespoonful), followed by gargling with a solution of half lemon juice and half water every hour during the waking hours for a day or two. In addition, a cotton swab may be used for applying the lemon juice directly to the tonsils several times a day. It will also help to apply some juice externally to the throat area of the neck.

The symptoms of influenza may often be relieved by drinking lemon juice with an equal amount of water three or four times a day.

Running of secretions from the nose, throat or head can usually be stopped by taking a tablespoonful of lemon juice several times a day. In addition, a solution of half lemon juice and half water should be sniffed into the nostrils twice daily, in the morning and at night.

The juice of the lemon is also useful in reducing obesity. Reports indicate that the juice of one-half lemon in a cup of warm water before breakfast will assist the body in the digestion of food and tend to prevent accumulation of fatty deposits.

Case histories indicate that lemon juice, taken in large quantities, is helpful in cases of liver ailments, asthma, colds, fevers, headaches, pneumonia, rheumatism, arthritis, neuritis, and many other conditions where Vitamin C is a factor in correcting vitamin deficiencies.

Preparation: This fruit is invaluable in the kitchen; its versatility ranges from simple sprinkling on fish or a freshly steamed vegetable to being a main ingredient in such lavish sauces as hollandaise or a Brazilian pepper and lemon sauce.

Two recipes made with lemons that children love are lemon chiffon custard and lemon cookies. To make the custard, first take one and one-half tablespoons gelatin and soak in one-half cup cold water. Place one pint hot water, four tablespoons lemon juice and four tablespoons honey in a double boiler over boiling water. Beat four egg yolks and slowly pour the hot water, lemon juice and honey into the eggs, stirring the mixture until set. Add one teaspoon vanilla extract and gelatin and stir briskly for two minutes. When cool and custard begins to set, beat with an eggbeater until smooth and thick. Place in refrigerator for several hours. Serve with whipped cream flavored with honey and vanilla, and garnish with grated lemon rind.

In this recipe oranges may be substituted for the lemons, both equally delicious and nourishing, making this a perfect treat for children. To make the cookies, take one-half cup honey and blend with one-half cup oil; blend with three tablespoons orange rind, three tablespoons lemon rind and one tablespoon lemon juice (or orange juice). Beat in one egg yolk, which has been slightly beaten, and two and one-half cups whole wheat flour, one-half cup wheat germ, and one-quarter cup ground or finely chopped nuts. This batter should be stiff; if not, add more flour. Roll out and cut into rounds or any desired shape. Brush tops with egg white and sprinkle with more nuts. Arrange on oiled cookie sheet. Bake at 350 degrees until light brown, about ten minutes.

An unusual soup recipe from Greece is made quickly by placing one and one-half quarts stock (the rich extract of soluble parts of meat, fish or poultry) in a pot and heating until it boils. Stir in one-half cup raw brown rice, cover pot and simmer for thirty minutes. Mix one-quarter teaspoon savory with three tablespoons nutritional yeast and four eggs that have been beaten. Add the juice and grated rind of one lemon to the egg mixture and stir again. Gradually add one-half cup of hot stock to the egg mixture, stirring constantly. Remove pot from heat and add egg mixture to soup. Garnish with minced chives if desired, and serve.

Lemon is a perfect substitute for vinegar in salads, being more nourishing; it also is not irritating to the sensitive stomach lining. To make lemon French salad dressing, combine one-half cup olive or salad oil with one-half cup lemon juice, one-half teaspoon salt, a few grains of cayenne, and two tablespoons of honey, and shake well. A variation of this can be made with the addition of two tablespoons each of cream cheese and chopped ginger, beaten into the basic recipe.

A unique sauce for cooked meat or raw fish is the Brazilian pepper and lemon sauce. Combine four Tabasco peppers, drained, with one chopped onion, one clove garlic, one-half cup lemon juice, and a sprinkle of salt and freshly ground pepper. Cover and refrigerate until ready to use.

An extremely simple and delicious spread for fish or vegetables is made by taking one-half cup softened butter and blending with one tablespoon lemon rind that has been grated, one-half teaspoon minced basil, one-half teaspoon minced chervil, one teaspoon minced chives, and one tablespoon minced parsley. This will make about three-quarters cup of spread.

Lemon sherbet is a great treat for everyone and so easy to make. Mix one cup honey with three-quarter cup lemon juice and one-eighth teaspoon salt; add slowly to three cups milk and one cup cream. Pour into freezer can and freeze, using eight parts ice to one part salt. This makes one and one-half quarts.

LENTILS

Botanical information: Lentil seeds, small, round and flattish, are found in the pods of the bean family plant, *Lentilla lens*, of the family *Fabacea.*

Nutritive values:

Vitamin A: 570 I.U. per 100 gm.

Vitamin B: Thiamine .56 mg.; Riboflavin .24 mg.; Niacin 2.2 mg.

Vitamin C: 5 mg.

Protein: 25 gm.

Calories: 337

Fat: 1 gm.

Carbohydrates: 59.5 gm.

Calcium: 59 mg.

Iron: 7.4 mg.

Phosphorus: 423 mg.

Reported health benefits: This is a very nourishing food and a good body builder. They are very rich in the vital minerals and are recommended in cases of low blood pressure, anemia, and emaciation. Lentil soup is good for cases of ulcerated stomachs and ulcerated digestive tracts.

Preparation: Lentils are a staple food throughout most of the world. Highly nutritious, this legume is a good source of proteins for vegetarians. Prepared in a variety of ways, a favorite is lentil soup. Wash two cups of lentils and soak overnight in cold water. Drain, add three quarts of cold water and a three pound brisket of beef or hambone. Heat to boiling and simmer for two hours. Add one-half cup diced celery and cook another two hours, or until meat and lentils are tender. Remove meat and skim fat from stock. Saute one small onion that has been sliced in two tablespoons of fat. Add two tablespoons flour, two teaspoons salt and one-quarter teaspoon pepper, blend, add one cup stock gradually, cook until thick and smooth, then add remaining stock. If desired, you may add one cup tomatoes.

A delicious rice-lentil combination, known as Kedgeree in east India, is made by taking two tablespoons oil and heating in a large pot; saute one chopped onion and one clove minced garlic. Add one and one-half quarts stock, two bay leaves, one-half teaspoon ground cinnamon, twelve ground cardamom seeds, one-fourth teaspoon ground mace, six whole cloves, and one cup of lentils that have been soaked overnight. Cover and simmer for one and one-half hours; add one cup raw rice and simmer for an additional thirty minutes. Drain off any remaining liquid and steam mixture until rice is dry and fluffy.

Spanish lentils are made with three cups cooked lentils. Add two cups stewed tomatoes, three tablespoons oil, one chopped onion, one chopped green pepper, one teaspoon flour, one teaspoon salt, one teaspoon each of oregano and ground celery seeds; cover and simmer until thoroughly heated.

For a lentil loaf, take two and one-half cups cooked lentils and combine with one cup cooked millet, one beaten egg, two slices chopped, broiled bacon, two onions which have been grated, one clove minced garlic, one-half teaspoon salt, one-quarter cup parsley, one-quarter teaspoon thyme, and a pinch of nutmeg. Blend these ingredients together with enough stock to moisten; turn into oiled loaf pan and bake at three hundred and seventy-five degrees for forty to forty-five minutes. Serve with your favorite sauce.

LETTUCE, HEAD

Botanical information: Botanical name is scariola *(Linne)*. Genus: *Lactuca.* The cabbage head variety is known as *capitata* (Linne).

Nutritive values:

Vitamin A: 540 I.U. per 100 gm.	Fat: .2 gm.
Vitamin B: Thiamine .04 mg.; Riboflavin .08 mg.; Niacin .2 mg.	Carbohydrates: 2.9 gm.
	Calcium: 22 mg.
Vitamin C: 8 mg.	Iron: .5 mg.
Protein: 1.2 gm.	Phosphorus: 25 mg.
Calories: 15	Potassium: 125 mg.

Reported health benefits: The minerals and vitamins of lettuce have been found valuable for conditions such as anemia, constipation, insomnia, nervousness, catarrh, tuberculosis, obesity, circulatory diseases, gout, poor appetite, urinary tract diseases, rheumatism and arthritis. There is a substantial amount of Vitamin E found in lettuce, especially in the Romaine variety, which contains more vitamins and minerals than head (iceberg) lettuce. The high percentage of iron in lettuce makes this food desirable for anemic conditions.

Preparation: Lettuce is commonly used as a side dish with the noon and evening meals. For those who enjoy vegetable soups, one and one-half cups of shredded lettuce may be mixed with one-half cup tomatoes and cooked for half an hour or until tender with two medium sized sliced onions, a cup of chopped celery, a cup of chopped beet tops, and with several herb spices added for flavoring.

LIME

Botanical information: Known as *citrus medica acida* of the family *Rutacae.*

Nutritive values:

	Calories: 37
Vitamin B: Thiamine .04 mg.;	Fat: .1 gm.
Riboflavin, trace; Niacin .1 mg.	Calcium: 40 mg.
Vitamin C: 27 mg.	Iron: .6 mg.
Protein: .8 gm.	Phosphorus: 22 mg.

Reported health benefits: The high Vitamin C content and other vitamins and minerals makes the lime valuable for cases of arthritis, scurvy and some liver ailments. The lime may be used as an antiseptic in the same manner as the lemon.

Preparation: Lime juice may be substituted in recipes where lemon juice is mentioned.

Lime or lemon juice may be used for a healthful French dressing to use with vegetable salads. Take one-half cup of either lime or lemon juice and mix with one-half cup of pure olive oil and two tablespoons of honey. Add a pinch of salt to taste and a few grains of cayenne. By combining all ingredients, this will make a cup of French dressing.

Lime or lemon juice may be used freely with herb teas to add to the flavor of the tea. Of course, if sweetness is desired, honey may be added.

LOGANBERRY

Botanical information: This is a hybrid plant resulting from crossing the red Antwerp raspberry with a species of blackberry. (Judge Logan, originator.)

Nutritive values:

Vitamin A: 200 I.U. per 100 gm.

Vitamin B: Thiamine .03 mg.; Riboflavin .04 mg.; Niacin .4 mg.

Vitamin C: 24 mg.

Proteins: 1.0 gm.

Calories: 62

Fat: .6 gm.

Carbohydrates: 14.9 gm.

Calcium: 35 mg.

Iron: 1.2 mg.

Phosphorus: 17 mg.

Reported health benefits: The medicinal values of the loganberry are similar to the values of the blackberry and the raspberry (see appropriate sections).

Preparation: Loganberries, after washing (rinsing), make a delicious dessert or may be used as a side dish with any meal. They may be added to breakfast cereals and, if sweetening is desired, some honey may be spread over the berries.

LOQUAT

Botanical information: Fruit of the tree known as *Eriobotrya japonica,* a native of eastern Asia, but also cultivated in some of the southern states.

Nutritive values:

Vitamin A: 670 I.U. per 100 gms.

Vitamin B: None

Vitamin C: 36 mg.

Protein: .9 gm.

Calories: 65

Fat: .1 gm.

Carbohydrates: 17.1 gm.

Calcium: 63 mg.

Iron: .4 mg.

Phosphorus: 42 mg.

Reported health benefits: Studies indicate that the loquat is beneficial for cases of constipation, obesity, acidosis, and a general body purification food.

Preparation: This fruit is best eaten very ripe, uncooked. It may be added to fruit salads, or blended with other fruits to make a delicious fruit drink.

LYCHEE NUTS

Botanical information: Also spelled Litchi, is the most celebrated fruit of China of the tree *Litchi clunenses.*

Nutritive values (per 100 gm.):

FRESH	DRIED
Vitamin A: none	none
Vitamin B: Riboflavin .05 mg.	none
Vitamin C: 42 mg.	none
Protein: .9 gm.	3.8 gm.
Calories 64	277
Fat: .3 gm.	1.2 gm.
Carbohydrates: 16.4 gm.	70.7 gm.
Calcium: 8 mg.	33 mg.
Iron: .4 mg.	1.7 mg.
Phosphorus: 43 mg.	181 mg.

Reported health benefits: There are no reported health benefits of the lychee nut other than the general benefits of its nutrients.

Preparation: Serve fresh lychee nuts for eating out of hand. They are even interesting to peel, or peel, chill and serve in a small sherbet dish garnished with a sprig of mint.

If you are using lychee nuts in combination with other fruits, the tropical ones such as pineapple, papayas, bananas and mangoes are the best.

The dried lychee nuts are soaked, boiled, and then added to rice dishes, stuffing, or combined in vegetable casseroles.

MACADAMIA

Botanical information: Any Australian tree of the genus *Macadamia,* especially the *ternifolia.*

Nutritive values:

Vitamin B: Thiamine .34 mg.; Riboflavin .11 mg.; Niacin 1.3 mg.
Protein: 7.8 gm.
Calories: 691
Fat: 71.6 gm.
Carbohydrates: 15.9 gm.
Calcium: 48 mg.
Iron: 2.0 mg.
Phosphorus: 161 mg.

Reported health benefits: The macadamia nut is unusual in that it contains not only protein, fat and a large number of calories and carbohydrates, but also contains a large supply of calcium, phosphorus and iron. It is an excellent food for body building and conditions of anemia and weakness, especially for convalescence.

Preparation: They may be eaten raw or ground and mixed with other foods.

MAMEY

Botanical information: Fruit of the tropical American tree *mammea americana*. Pomelo-like in size and shape.

Nutritive values:

Vitamin A: 230 I.U. per 100 gm. Fat: .5 gm.
Vitamin B: Thiamine .02 mg.; Carbohydrates: 12.5 gm.
  Riboflavin .04 mg.; Niacin .4 mg. Calcium: 11 mg.
Vitamin C: 14 mg. Iron: .7 mg.
Protein: .5 gm. Phosphorus: 11 mg.
Calories: 51

Reported health benefits: This exotic tropical plant contains practically all of the vitamins and minerals and would be excellent for obesity and ailments of the heart, liver and kidney that usually accompany obesity.

Preparation: May be eaten raw as a delicious fruit or it may be added to a salad of other fruits and vegetables.

MANGO

Botanical information: The mango is the fruit of *Mangifera indica*. It is esteemed as one of the most delicious tropical fruits.

Nutritive values:

Vitamin A: 6,350 I.U. per 100 gm. Fat: .2 gm.
Vitamin B: Thiamine .06 mg.; Calcium: 9 mg.
  Riboflavin .06 mg.; Niacin .9 mg. Iron: .2 mg.
Vitamin C: 41 mg. Phosphorus: 13 mg.
Protein: .7 gm.
Calories: 66

Reported health benefits: This fruit is reported to be beneficial for inflammation of the kidneys (nephritis) as well as for other kidney ailments. This fruit is also valuable to combat acidity and poor digestion. It has also been found to be helpful in reducing fevers and for respiratory ailments. It is helpful in relieving clogged pores of the skin and has been found valuable in relieving cases of inflammation of bladder-like sacs in the body known as cysts.

Preparation: This delicious fruit may be used simply as a delicious fruit to be eaten between meals or after meals. It may be cut into small portions and used as a side dish or added to cereals for flavoring.

MILLET

Botanical information: *Panicum miliaceum.* This is the seed of a grass widely cultivated for use as a cereal in Europe.

Nutritive values:

Vitamin B: Thiamine .73 mg.; Riboflavin .38 mg.; Niacin 2.3 mg.
Protein: 9.9 gm.
Calories: 327
Fat: 2.9 gm.
Carbohydrates: 72.9 gm.
Calcium: 20 mg.
Iron: 6.8 mg.
Phosphorus: 311 mg.

Reported health benefits: Millet is easily digested, having a low starch content. It is a valuable food for constipation, and also beneficial for weight gain and general emaciation

Preparation: Millet is a popular breakfast food. It cooks quickly and is extremely nutritious, especially with the addition of sunflower seeds, dried fruits, etc. It may be used in baking, replacing sunflower or sesame seeds; also, ground into a meal, it may be sprinkled over other foods.

MUNG BEAN SPROUTS

Botanical information: The mung bean or moong bean is a species of the kidney bean. It is a plant of the genus *phaseolus vulgaris.*

Nutritive values:

Vitamin A: 10 I.U. per 100 gm.
Vitamin B: Thiamine .07 mg.; Riboflavin .09 mg.; Niacin .5 mg.
Vitamin C: 15 mg.
Protein: 2.9 gm.
Calories: 23
Fat: .2 gm.
Carbohydrates: 4 1 gm.
Calcium: 29 mg.
Iron: .8 mg.
Phosphorus: 59 mg.
Potassium: 500 mg.

Reported health benefits: Sprouts do much to relieve malnutrition and to eliminate toxic poisons from the system. This is done mainly by providing the body with the nutrients needed and nature does the work of restoration. The many vitamins and minerals in sprouts are at their highest peak of activity while sprouting, and absorption into the body at this time is of maximum benefit. They have been found valuable for arthritis, neuritis, rheumatism, constipation, and many other chronic ailments.

Preparation: Sprouts may be eaten alone or placed in a blender and blended with various juices for a more nutritious drink. A popular use of sprouts is to mix them into an egg omelet.

MUSHROOM

Botanical information: The mushroom is a rapidly growing fungus of the class *Basidio mycetes* and order *Agaricales*.

Nutritive values:

Vitamin B: Thiamine .10 mg.; Riboflavin .44 mg.; Niacin 4.9 mg.
Vitamin C: 5 mg.
Protein: 2.4 gm.
Calories: 16

Fat: .3 gm.
Carbohydrates: 4 gm.
Calcium: 9 gm.
Iron: 1 mg.
Phosphorus: 115 mg.
Potassium: 150 mg.

Reported health benefits: There are no special health benefits for mushrooms other than the benefits ordinarily derived from the many vitamins and minerals found in this food.

Preparation: Mushrooms are prepared in many forms. They are baked, broiled and creamed, as well as used with other foods. They are popular with eggs made into omelets or scrambled. They are often combined with other foods into sandwiches and are popular in soups.

A good cream of mushroom soup is prepared by washing and skinning one-quarter pound of mushrooms and simmering the skins in one-half cup of water. The mushroom caps and stems should be chopped into small pieces and two cups of water added to the skins. The simmering should continue until the skins are tender. Melt two tablespoons of butter, adding two tablespoons whole wheat or soybean flour and one teaspoon salt. (Salt may be omitted when anyone is on a salt-free diet.) Two cups of milk should be added gradually over a low flame, stirring constantly until the soup thickens. The chopped mushroom should then be added, and when ready to serve add chopped parsley.

MUSTARD GREENS

Botanical information: From the family *Brassicaceae*.

Nutritive values:

Vitamin A: 6,460 I.U. per 100 gm.   Fat: .3 gm.
Vitamin B: Thiamine .09 mg.;   Carbohydrates: 4 gm.
  Riboflavin .20 mg.; Niacin .8 mg.   Calcium: 220 mg.
Vitamin C: 102 mg.   Iron: 2.9 mg.
Protein: 2.3 gm.   Phosphorus: 38 mg.
Calories: 22   Potassium: 500 mg.

Reported health benefits: This vegetable is recognized as an excellent tonic. It is valued for anemia, constipation, rheumatism, arthritis, acidity, kidney and bladder ailments, and inflammation of bronchial tubes (bronchitis). It is also valuable to pregnant women and for nursing mothers, and it is useful in ridding the system of poisonous substances. It is used as a counter-irritant or as an ingredient of mustard plasters and stimulating liniments.

Preparation: The leaves of the mustard green plant are popular as a salad leaf as part of the luncheon or dinner meal. It may also be placed into a blender and blended with fruit juices into a nutritious drink. It makes an excellent addition to soups. For cooked mustard greens, wash thoroughly in warm and cold water, place the leaves in a pan without water for ten to fifteen minutes on low heat, and cover tightly to prevent release of steam for cooked mustard greens.

NECTARINES

Botanical information: This variety of the peach differs from the common peach mainly in its smooth, waxy skin and a more fragrant pulp.

Nutritive values:

Vitamin A: 1,650 I.U. per 100 gm.   Fat: trace
                                           Carbohydrate: 17.1 gm.
Vitamin C: 13 mg.   Calcium: 4 mg.

Protein: .6 gm.
Calories: 64

Iron: .5 mg.
Phosphorus: 24 mg.

Reported health benefits: This fruit is valuable as a digestive aid and for relief of abdominal gas. It has also been recommended for high blood pressure, asthma and rheumatism, and will give relief for bladder ailments. Obese persons will find that generous use of nectarines will help to lose weight.

Preparation: This fruit is delicious as a dessert and is preferred in the raw state. It may be cut up with other fruits and served as a fruit salad, or it may be cooked slightly with other fruits and made into a compote.

OATS

Botanical information: The edible grain of the cereal grass *Avena sativa.*
Nutritive values:

Vitamin B: Thiamine .48 mg.;
    Riboflavin .11 mg.; Niacin .8 mg.
Protein: 11.4 gm.
Calories: 312
Fat: 5.9 gm.

Carbohydrates: 54.6 gm.
Calcium: 42 mg.
Iron: 3.6 mg.
Phosphorus: 324 mg.

Reported health benefits: Oats have been recommended as a general body builder and for muscle development. They are also said to help the glands, teeth, hair and nails. In some cases, there may be a constipating effect due to fermentation and gas. Oats also contain Vitamin E, said to be helpful for the heart.

Preparation: Oatmeal is usually served as a breakfast cereal with milk and honey, or with the addition of raisins and other fruits. However, it also may be used in baking. There are many delicious recipes for oatmeal bread, cookies and muffins.

OKRA

Botanical information: *Hibiscus* or *Abelmoschus esculentus*, native to Africa but cultivated in warm climates for the young mucilaginous pods.

Nutritive values:

Vitamin A: 740 I.U. per 100 gm.

Fat: Small trace.

Vitamin B: Small traces of B_1 (Thiamine) and B_2 (Riboflavin). Contains .8 mg. of B_3 (Niacin).
Vitamin C: 20 mg.
Protein: 1 gm.
Calories: 32

Carbohydrates: 7 gm.
Calcium: 82 mg.
Iron: .7 mg.
Phosphorus: 62 mg.
Potassium: 370 mg.

Reported health benefits: The mucilaginous nature of this vegetable makes okra suitable for treatment of stomach ulcers. It has also been found to be valuable for cases of inflammation of the lungs (pleurisy) and of the colon (colitis). It will also help in sore throat conditions, and when taken regularly will help to reduce excessive weight.

Preparation: Okra is delicious when cooked or added to vegetable soup. For cooking okra, wash the vegetable and cut off stems. Cut into half-inch slices and place in a saucepan. Add three-quarters teaspoon of salt and cover with water, and cook without covering for fifteen minutes or until soft enough to chew with comfort. Drain and serve, seasoning with pepper, butter and vinegar. The drained water is palatable and contains vitamins and minerals. For more effective medicinal purposes, the okra should be run through a juicer and the juice used for drinking and/or gargling for sore throat.

OLIVE

Botanical information: The evergreen tree *Olea europaea*, or the American olive tree *Osmanthus Americanus* of the South Atlantic coast, or in California, *Umbellularia Californica*.

Nutritive values:

Vitamin A: 300 I.U. per 100 gm.
Vitamin B: Trace of Thiamine only.

Protein: 1.5 gm.
Calories: 132

Fat: 13.5 gm.
Carbohydrates: 4.0 gm.
Calcium: 87 mg.
Iron: 1.6 mg.
Phosphorus: 17 mg.

Reported health benefits: Olive oil has been found to stimulate contractions of the gall bladder, and is therefore valuable for many kinds of gall bladder ailments. Olives will help liver disorders and have been reported as helpful in cases of diabetes, abdominal gas and indigestion problems. Olive oil will help to strengthen and develop body tissue and is highly rated as a tonic for the nerves. It will also relieve cases of constipation. The oil is also good for sunburn or other burns, as well as for minor skin eruptions and inflammations.

Preparation: Because of the improved flavor of foods, the addition of the oil of olives is a common practice. Olive oil is commonly a part of salad dressings and, in addition, chopped olives are used as a part of the dressing or chopped or whole olives are used as side dishes with all meals. A good salad dressing is to mix equal parts of olive oil and lemon juice, adding some honey for sweetening.

ONION

Botanical information: Known as *Allium cepa* of the family *Liliaceae*.

Nutritive values:

Vitamin A: 50 I.U. per 100 gm.	Fat: .2 gm.
Vitamin B: Thiamine .03 mg.;	Carbohydrates: 10.3 gm.
Riboflavin .04 mg.; Niacin .2 mg.	Calcium: 32 mg.
Vitamin C: 9 mg.	Iron: .5 mg.
Protein: 1.4 gm.	Phosphorus: 44 mg.
Calories: 45	Potassium: 300 mg.

Reported health benefits: Onions increase the flow of urine, are slightly laxative and have antiseptic qualities. For sinus conditions, they help to drain mucus from the cavities and loosen phlegm. Onions have been found valuable for the hair, nails of the fingers and toes, and for the eyes. They have also been recommended for cases of asthma (difficult breathing), bronchitis (inflammation of the bronchial tubes), pneumonia, influenza and colds. Victims of tuberculosis have been known to improve following a heavy consumption of onions. This vegetable has also improved cases of low blood pressure, insomnia, neuritis (inflammation of nerves), vertigo (dizziness), and obesity. It will also help destroy worms and other parasites in the body. A poultice of crushed onions applied to the chest has been reported to relieve cases of inflammation of the lungs (pleurisy) and a poultice of crushed onions is reported to relieve boils on the skin.

Preparation: Onions are commonly used with many foods. They are popular in the preparation of scalloped potatoes and are prepared with scrambled eggs and as egg omelets. For scalloped eggs with onions, sliced onions are combined with sliced hard-boiled eggs in alternate layers in an oiled baking dish. Baking in a moderate oven for approximately one hour is sufficient to make the onions tender.

Another good onion casserole dish is to first parboil (half-boil) several peeled onions in boiling water for about five minutes, and then drain out the water and place the onions in a casserole dish. Combine an equal amount of honey and tomatoes (or tomato catchup) and pour over the onions. Some butter may be placed into the casserole dish for flavoring, and some herbs and spices may be sprinkled over the dish just prior to baking in a moderate oven of 375°F. for forty-five minutes or until the onions are tender.

While fresh spring green onions may be eaten raw in a vegetable salad, the onions may be trimmed and cooked in boiling salted water until tender. A popular sauce for spreading over cooked onions and other vegetables (Hollandaise sauce) is made by melting one-half cup butter and adding two egg yolks into the butter, one at a time, blending each yolk into the butter thoroughly. Add one-quarter teaspoon salt and a dash of cayenne pepper and beat well. Just before serving, add one-half cup of boiling water gradually into the mixture, beating constantly. Cook over hot water, stirring constantly until thickened, and serve at once.

ORANGE

Botanical information: The botanical name of the orange is *Citrus aurantium.* Favorite varieties are the mandarin orange of China, the California navel orange and the tangerine.

Nutritive values:

Vitamin A: 190

Vitamin B: Thiamine .08 mg.;
  Riboflavin .03 mg.; Niacin .2 mg.

Vitamin C: 49 mg.

Protein: .9 gm.

Calories: 45

Fat: .2 gm.

Carbohydrates: 11.2 gm.

Calcium: 33 mg.

Iron: .4 mg.

Phosphorus: 23 mg.

Potassium: 300 mg.

Reported health benefits: Oranges have been recommended to help overcome many ailments, including asthma, bronchitis, tuberculosis, pneumonia, rheumatism, arthritis and high blood pressure. Persons addicted to alcohol have found that the desire for liquor is greatly reduced by the drinking of orange juice. Others suffering from obesity have been able to reduce hunger pangs and food cravings by ample partaking of oranges. Consumption of large quantities of oranges will decrease the outpouring of mucus secretions from the nose and head. While in some cases oranges may bring about skin eruptions, this is probably due to poisonous substances in the body being driven out by the effect of the oranges. Eventually, the eruptions will cease after the toxins have been eliminated. However, oranges or orange juice should not be consumed in cases of stomach ulcers or inflammation of the stomach or intestines.

Preparation: The most popular form of eating the orange is by peeling it and eating it section by section or by drinking juice squeezed from the orange. However, it is often frequently eaten as a dessert, the sections of the fruit being placed in a bowl with other fruits such as the apple, pear, pineapple, etc. Orange juice is often added to recipes for bread, cake, and fillings for extra flavor, and is a favorite ingredient for pies, puddings, ice cream, sherbet, sauces and custards.

The orange peel may be eaten raw and is reported to be a digestive aid. It is a favorite candy for children as well as grown-ups when the peel is cut into thin strips about one-quarter inch wide and boiled for fifteen minutes with a teaspoonful of salt. The water is then discarded and fresh water is added for an additional boiling of about twenty minutes. The water is then changed a third time, the peel boiled again for twenty minutes, and the peel strips drained thoroughly. Assuming the use of six orange shells, the strips may then be dipped in honey and are then ready for serving. The orange peel candy has been recommended for relieving acid conditions of the stomach and intestines, and will relieve diarrhea conditions.

PAPAW

Botanical information: Fruit of the tropical American tree *carica papaya.*

Nutritive values:

No Vitamins or Minerals	Fat: .2 gm.
Protein: 5.2 gm.	Carbohydrates: 16.8 gm.
Calories: 85	

Preparation: The juice of the fruit or leaves is applied in various ways as an excellent meat tenderizer.

PAPAYA

Botanical information: Fruit of the *papaw tree (Carica papaya)*.

Nutritive values:

Vitamin A: 1,750 I.U. per 100 gm.   Fat: .1 gm.
Vitamin B: Thiamine .03 mg.;   Carbohydrates: 10 gm.
   Riboflavin .04 mg.; Niacin .3 mg.   Calcium: 20 mg.
Vitamin C: 56 mg.   Iron: .3
Protein: .6 gm.   Phosphorus: 16 mg.
Calories: 39   Potassium: 470 mg.

Reported health benefits: This fruit contains the digestive enzyme *papain* and is therefore valuable for aiding digestion. It is easily digestible and cleanses the digestive tract. Case studies indicate that this food, taken alone for two or three days, has a highly beneficial tonic effect upon the stomach and intestines. The juice of the papaya aids in relieving infections in the colon and has a tendency to break down pus and mucus reached by the juice. Leaves of the papaya tree have been found valuable as a dressing for ulcerated wounds. This fruit also contains Vitamins D, E and K.

Preparation: The fruit can be eaten raw, cooked or pickled, and juice of the squeezed fruit makes an excellent drink. An excellent salad is prepared by cutting the meat of the papaya into slices or small pieces and mixing with other fruits or vegetables, and served on crisp lettuce leaves.

PARSLEY

Botanical information: A biennial plant known as *Petroselinum*.

Nutritive values:

Vitamin A: 8,230 I.U. per 100 gm.   Fat: 1.0 gm.
Vitamin B: Thiamine .11 mg.;   Carbohydrates: 9.0 gm.
   Riboflavin .28 mg.; Niacin 1.4   Calcium: 193 mg.
   mg.   Iron: 4.3 mg.
Vitamin C: 193 mg.   Phosphorus: 84 mg.
Protein: 3.7 gm.   Potassium: 80 mg.
Calories: 50   Copper and manganese are
                                also present.

Reported health benefits: The richness of minerals in parsley as well as the high content of vitamins has made parsley valuable for cases of anemia, nephritis (inflammation of the kidneys), tuberculosis, halitosis, menstruation disorders, fevers, dropsy (accumulation of fluid in a cavity), congested liver and gall bladder, diseases of the urinary tract, rheumatism, arthritis, acidosis (deficiency of alkaline in the body), obesity, high blood pressure, catarrh (discharge from inflammed mucous membrane), dyspepsia (difficult digestion), and in treatment of venereal diseases.

Preparation: Parsley may be converted into a juice with the aid of a fruit and vegetable juicer, and drinking of parsley juice has been found valuable in removing poisonous drugs from the body. It has also proved to be effective in dissolving kidney or other stones of the body when taken raw in juice form.

Parsley should always be eaten raw for preservation of the food value.

It is useful to chew it for removing onion and garlic odors from the breath.

When prepared as a tea with about one-quarter teaspoon of powdered parsley to the cup, parsley tea has been found to be helpful for diabetes cases. It is also a mild sedative and a diuretic when taken as a tea. When parsley flakes are used, about one-half teaspoonful to a cup of boiling water would be a suitable amount.

While raw parsley retains the full food value, chopped parsley may be added to soups as a garnish or for seasoning. In addition, a healthful broth may be prepared by simmering a cupful of chopped parsley with either tomatoes or potatoes. For persons ill or convalescing from illness, the broth, after simmering for about twenty minutes, may be strained and then served with a small quantity of whole milk and butter.

PARSNIP

Botanical information: *Pastinaca sativa* of the family *Apiaceae.*

Nutritive values:

Vitamin B: Thiamine .08 mg.;
    Riboflavin .12 mg.; Niacin .2 mg.
Vitamin C: 18 mg.
Protein: 1.5 gm.
Calories: 78

Fat: .5 gm.
Carbohydrates: 18.2 gm.
Calcium: 57 gm.
Iron: .7 mg.
Phosphorus: 80 mg.
Potassium: 570 mg.

Reported health benefits: Recommended for gout (inflammation of joints), tuberculosis, colitis (inflammation of the colon), neuritis (inflammation of a nerve), insomnia, hemorrhoids, diarrhea, stomach ulcers, and as a diuretic for increasing the secretion of urine. Parsnips tend to remove toxins from the kidney apparatus as well as kidney stones.

Preparation: Parsnips may be boiled, steamed or baked. The cooking should be done quickly in the minimum time necessary for the parsnips to become soft enough to chew, usually from eight to ten minutes.

Parsnips may also be converted into a juice and when taken frequently in this form will usually give prompt relief for brittle nails and mild nervous disorders.

PEACH

Botanical information: *Prunus* or *Amygdalus persica.*

Nutritive values:

Vitamin A: 880 I.U. per 100 gm.   Fat: .1 gm.
Vitamin B: Thiamine: .02 mg.;   Carbohydrates: 12 gm.
   Riboflavin .05 mg.; Niacin .9 mg.   Calcium: 8 mg.
Vitamin C: 8 mg.   Iron: .6 mg.
Protein: .5 gm.   Phosphorus: 22 mg.
Calories: 46   Potassium: 310 mg.

Reported health benefits: The vitamins and minerals in peaches have made this tasty fruit valuable for anemia, constipation, high blood pressure, gastritis (inflammation of the stomach), nephritis (inflammation of the kidneys), acidosis (deficiency of alkalinity in the body), bronchitis (inflammation of the bronchial tubes), asthma, difficult digestion, and for bladder and kidney stones. Peaches also help improve the health of the skin and add color to the complexion. They have also been reported as helpful in removal of worms from the intestinal tract.

Preparation: Peaches make excellent fruit salads when combined with such other fruits as apricots, apples, bananas, pineapples, pears, oranges and grapefruit, and placed over lettuce leaves. Peach halves filled with cottage cheese on a bed of crisp endives and garnished with ripe olives in the center of the cheese make a delicious and healthy salad.

PEANUTS

Botanical information: *Arachis hypogaiae* of the bean family.

Nutritive values:

Vitamin B: Thiamine .30 mg.; Riboflavin .13 mg.; Niacin 16.2 mg.

Protein: 26.9 gm.
Calories: 559

Fat: 44.2 gm.
Carbohydrates: 23.6 gm.
Calcium: 74 mg.
Iron: 1.9 mg.
Phosphorus: 393 mg.
Potassium: 337 mg.
Vitamin E: Amount undetermined.

Reported health benefits: The high protein and calorie value of peanuts, especially of peanut butter, makes this a nourishing and body-building food. The high fat content may make this food undesirable for persons over-supplied with fat but for persons suffering from under-weight, low blood pressure or general weakness, peanuts are very valuable.

Preparation: Peanuts may be eaten raw, boiled or roasted. They may be spread on desserts or salads, or made into peanut butter. With the use of a blender, peanuts may be blended into various fruit drinks, puddings or ice cream.

PEAR

Botanical information: *Pyrus communis* of the family *Pomaceae*.

Nutritive values:

Vitamin A: 20 I.U. per 100 gm.
Vitamin B: Thiamine .02 mg.; Riboflavin .04 mg.; Niacin .1 mg.
Vitamin C: 4 mg.
Protein: .7 gm.
Calories: 63

Fat: .4 gm.
Carbohydrates: 15.8 gm.
Calcium: 13 mg.
Iron: .3 mg.
Phosphorus: 16 mg.
Potassium: 182 mg.

Reported health benefits: This fruit is recommended for constipation and poor digestion, as well as for high blood pressure and obesity. It also helps the condition of nephritis (inflammation of the kidneys) and acidosis (deficiency in alkalinity of the body). It has been found helpful for skin conditions such as eruptions and inflamed conditions of the colon, known as colitis. Pears have been found to help cases of catarrh, where discharges from the mucous membranes occur.

Preparation: Pears are most nutritious when eaten fresh; however, they can be added to other fruits in a fruit salad, blended into fruit drinks or made into puddings, pies or ice creams.

PEAS, IMMATURE

Botanical information: The pea is the edible seed of the plant *Pisum sativum.*

Nutritive values:

Vitamin A: 680 I.U. per gm.
Vitamin B: Thiamine .34 mg.;
  Riboflavin .16 mg.; Niacin 2.7
  mg.
Vitamin C: 26 mg.
Protein: 6.7 gm.
Calories: 98

Fat: .4 gm.
Carbohydrates: 17.7 gm.
Calcium: 22 mg.
Iron: 1.9 mg.
Phosphorus: 122 mg.
Potassium: 200 mg.

Reported health benefits: Peas are excellent for nourishment and strength restoring and building. It is a good food for persons suffering from anemia, low blood pressure and who are underweight. Peas contain nicotinic acid, reportedly recommended for reducing cholesterol in the blood.

Preparation: There are many ways of preparing peas. The most popular method is to place in small pot, sprinkle lightly with various tasty herbs and spices, and then cover with boiling water. Allow to simmer only until tender.

Peas are often used as side dishes with various meat dishes. Another popular dish using peas is to combine with chopped parsley and chopped mint, using the parsley and mint to season and flavor the peas during the cooking process. A casserole dish with peas for serving eight persons is to take four cups of cooked peas and place them in a greased baking dish or casserole. One-quarter teaspoon of salt is sprinkled on the peas, followed by the addition of about one-eighth teaspoon of black pepper and one cup of whole milk. A cup of grated cheese already mixed with two tablespoons of minced pimento is then sprinkled over the top. Baking is done in a hot oven of 400° for about twenty minutes, or until cheese is melted.

Peas may also be cooked with lettuce. Several layers of washed lettuce leaves are placed in the bottom of a kettle and about two pounds of peas on the lettuce. Take several additional lettuce leaves and cover the peas. Cooking is done over low heat for twenty minutes. This is enough to serve four persons. When ready to serve, the peas and lettuce may be flavored with spices and garnished with mint sprigs.

PEAS, MATURE

Botanical information: *Pisum sativum.*

Nutritive values:

Vitamin A: 370 I.U. per 100 gm.
Vitamin B: Thiamine .77 mg.; Riboflavin .28 mg.; Niacin 3.1 mg.
Vitamin C: 2 mg.
Protein: 23.8 gm.
Calories: 339

Fat: 1.4 gm.
Carbohydrates: 60.2
Calcium: 57 mg.
Iron: 4.7 mg.
Phosphorus: 388 mg.
Potassium: 200 mg.

Reported health benefits: See the discussion of Peas, immature.

PECAN

Botanical information: Known as *Hicoria pecan.*

Nutritive values:

Vitamin A: 50 I.U. per 100 gm.
Vitamin B: Thiamine .72 mg.; Riboflavin .11 mg.; Niacin .9 mg.
Vitamin C: 2 mg.
Protein: 9.4 gm.
Calories: 696

Fat: 73 gm.
Carbohydrates: 13 gm.
Calcium: 74 mg.
Iron: 2.4 mg.
Phosphorus: 324 mg.
Potassium: 300 mg.

Reported health benefits: The pecan is a rich food and has been found valuable for cases of low blood pressure, general weakness and emaciation, and for persons needing nourishment for the teeth.

Preparation: The ideal method of eating pecans is to simply remove the outer shell and eat them raw. However, they can be included in recipes for bread, cookies, ice cream, pie, rolls or puddings.

PEPPER, GREEN

Botanical information: *Capsicum annum.*

Nutritive values:

Vitamin A: 630 I.U. per 100 gm.   Fat: .2 gm.
Vitamin B: Thiamine .04 mg.;   Carbohydrates: 5.7 gm.
   Riboflavin .07 mg.; Niacin .4 mg.   Calcium: 11 mg.
Vitamin C: 120 mg.   Iron: .4 mg.
Protein: 1.2 gm.   Phosphorus: 25 mg.
Calories: 25   Potassium: 170 mg.

Reported health benefits: The green pepper, bell-shaped, should be eaten raw for deriving maximum nourishment from the vitamins and minerals of this vegetable. Peppers are especially valuable for liver disorders, obesity, constipation, high blood pressure and acidosis (deficiency of alkalinity in the body). The smaller red peppers, known as hot peppers, have been found to be valuable for colds, asthma and inflamed sinuses. They have also been used with success in cases of malaria and for destroying intestinal wcrms. Because of their sharpness in taste, the red peppers should be avoided when there is any inflammation or tenderness of the stomach or intestinal tract.

Preparation: The large green peppers are ideal for stuffing with different foods such as meat, minced vegetables, tomatoes, cabbage, carrots, or almost any other foods. The stem and seeds are removed before stuffing the peppers.

PERSIMMONS

Botanical information: *Diospyros Virginiana* of the family *Ebenaceae.*

Nutritive values:

Vitamin A: 2,710 I.U. per 100 gm.   Fat: .4 gm.
Vitamin B: Thiamine .05 mg.;   Carbohydrates: 20 gm.
   Riboflavin .05 mg.; Niacin, trace.   Calcium: 6 mg.
Vitamin C: 11 mg.   Iron: .3 mg.
Protein: .8 gm.   Phosphorus: 26 mg.
Calories: 78   Potassium: 310 mg.

Reported health benefits: This is an excellent food for energy. It is also very soothing to the intestinal tract and therefore is of great value for cases of stomach or intestinal ulcers or other conditions requiring nourishment, without danger of injury to delicate mucous membrane such as constipation, colitis (infection of the colon) and hemorrhoids. Persimmons have also been recommended for pleurisy and sore throat conditions.

Preparation: The unripe green fruit has a high percentage of tannic and malic acid. The preferred way of drinking is to take three persimmons and cut them into small pieces. A cup of hot water is then poured over the fruit and allowed to steep for several minutes. When a strong solution is prepared, it may be used to aid cases of ulcerated or sore throats.

When fully mature, the fruit is deliciously sweet.

PIGNOLIA

Botanical information: The edible seed of the cones of a nut pine. *Pineus* of the pine.

Nutritive values:

Vitamin A: 230 I.U. per 100 gm.	Proteins: 31.1 gm.
Vitamin B: Thiamine .67 mg.;	Calories: 552
Riboflavin none; Niacin 1.4 mg.	Fat: 47.4 gm.
	Carbohydrates: 11.6 gm.

Reported health benefits: The pignolia, or pine nut as it is sometimes called, is one of the best sources of protein in the nut family. It has been found to be a good aid in nourishing and building a strong body for those suffering from emaciation. It is also recommended in cases of low blood pressure and run-down conditions.

Preparation: Pignolia nuts, like all other nuts, should be eaten raw; in this way they are more easily digested and the natural flavor is preserved.

Since pignolias are a soft nut, they need not be ground; however, it is still best to chew them well, making them more digestible. They can be added to salads, nut drinks, or just eaten plain.

Nuts are highly perishable, so it is best to keep them refrigerated until used.

PILINUT

Botanical information: The Pilinut (pronounced pee-lee-nut) is an edible seed of the Philippine burseraceous tree *Canarium ovatum*. The seed tastes like a sweet almond.

Nutritive values:

Vitamin A: 40 I.U. per 100 gm.

Vitamin B: Thiamine .88 mg.;
Riboflavin .09 mg.; Niacin .5 mg.

Vitamin C: trace

Protein: 11.4 gm.

Calories: 669

Fat: 71.1 gm.

Carbohydrates: 8.4 gm.

Calcium: 140 mg.

Iron: 3.4 mg.

Phosphorus: 554 mg.

Reported health benefits: The high content of calcium, phosphorus and iron, together with Vitamins A and B and the protein content and calorie value, makes this nut excellent for vitality, endurance, and the bone structure. It prevents and helps anemia problems and nourishes the brain and nerves. The phosphorus stimulates the growth of hair and bone.

Preparation: They may be eaten raw or ground and mixed with other foods or drinks.

PINE NUTS OR PINON NUTS

Botanical information: Pine nuts are seeds of any of several pine trees.

Nutritive values:

Vitamin A: 30 I.U. per 100 gm.

Vitamin B: Thiamine 1.28 mg.;
Riboflavin .23 mg.; Niacin 4.5 mg.

Vitamin C: trace

Protein: 13 gm.

Calories: 635

Fat: 60.5 gm.

Carbohydrates: 20.5 gm.

Calcium: 12 mg.

Iron: 5.2 mg.

Phosphorus: 604 mg.

Reported health benefits: The presence of Vitamins A and B, together with protein, fats, carbohydrates, calcium and iron, makes this an excellent food for body building, strength and energy. The high calorie content makes this highly desirable for active people.

Preparation· They may be eaten raw or ground and mixed with other foods.

PINEAPPLE

Botanical information: The pineapple is the fruit of the tropical plant *Ananas ananas.*

Nutritive values:

Vitamin A: 130 I.U. per 100 gm.	Fat: .2 gm.
Vitamin B: Thiamine .08 mg.;	Carbohydrates: 13.7 gm.
Riboflavin .02 mg.; Niacin .2.	Calcium: 16 mg.
Vitamin C: 24 mg.	Iron: .3 mg.
Protein: .4 gm.	Phosphorus: 11 mg.
Calories: 52	Potassium: 150 mg.

Reported health benefits: In addition to many vitamins and minerals, pineapples contain papain, which aids digestion, and chlorine, valuable for digestion of proteins. Pineapples are also good for constipation, and because of the aid to digestion help to rid the body of excess weight. This fruit is also esteemed as a regulator of the glands and has been found valuable for cases of goiter (enlargement of the thyroid gland), dyspepsia (chronic digestive disturbances), bronchitis (inflammation of the bronchial tubes), catarrh (secretions from mucous membranes), high blood pressure, arthritis (disease of the joints) and tumors.

Pineapple juice is widely used in some areas for expelling intestinal worms, but this applies only to the juice in natural form and not to the canned juice. Fresh pineapple has been used in order to combat diphtheria or other infections of the throat or other parts of the body.

Preparation: There are numerous ways of including pineapples into the diet, but of course the most simple and most beneficial way is to slice it, remove the peel and eat the fruit in its natural form. However, pineapple is often included in bread, cake and cookie recipes as well as in pies, puddings and salads. Slices of pineapple are often placed with slices of meat in sandwiches.

A delicious bread can be made with pineapple, honey and chopped nuts with whole wheat flour. A cup of honey is blended with two tablespoons of shortening, preferably 100 percent corn oil, and these two items are beaten together with one egg. Two cups of whole wheat flour and three teaspoons of baking powder are blended together with one-half teaspoon salt, together with one-half cup of chopped nuts. A cup of pure pineapple juice is added to the egg and shortening mix, and all ingredients are gradually mixed together and then poured into a greased loaf pan and baked in a moderate oven of approximately 325° for about one and one-quarter hours.

A delightful fresh pineapple pie may be made by beating two eggs slightly with a cup of brown sugar, a tablespoonful of lemon juice, and two cups of shredded fresh pineapple. The pie pan may then be lined with graham crackers and the mixture poured into the pan. It will take only about ten minutes to bake this pineapple pie in a very hot oven of 450°, after which it should be baked for thirty-five minutes in a moderate oven of 350° or until the pineapple is tender.

Lovely pineapple baskets are served by cutting a pineapple into halves lengthwise and scooping out the pulp in cubes or balls. The pineapple scoops are then mixed with other fruits such as strawberries, apple pieces or sections of pear, orange, melon, or other fruits in season.

PISTACHIO

Botanical information: Nut of a small Asian tree *(Pistacia vera)*

Nutritive values:

Vitamin A: 230 I.U. per 100 gm.

Vitamin B: Thiamine .22 mg.; Riboflavin .11 mg.; Niacin .7 mg.

Protein: 19.3 gm.

Fat: 53;7 gm.

Calories: 594

Fat: 53.7 gm.

Carbohydrates: 19.0 gm.

Reported health benefits: This nut is recommended in cases of low blood pressure and low vitality. It aids in the proper development of teeth and bones, and is a general body builder.

Preparation: Avoid the commercial dyed and salted nuts that are sold in many food stores. Most health food stores carry the pistachio nuts that have been roasted slightly, with or without the addition of sea salt. These can be enjoyed right from the shell. They are very nutritious, a good energy food, and fairly easily digested. The reason that many people believe nuts to be undigestible is that they eat them after a heavy meal, including heavy desserts. The dessert is the culprit and not the nuts. It is important, however, that nuts be chewed thoroughly for proper digestion, as the digestive juices cannot break down the tough kernels.

PITANGA

Botanical information: Fruit of the South American tree, *malpighia glabra,* also grown in Florida and California. Also known as the Surinam cherry.

Nutritive values:

Vitamin A: 1500 I.U. per 100 gm.	Fat: .4 gm.
Vitamin B: Thiamine .03 mg.;	Carbohydrates: 12.5 gm.
Riboflavin .04 mg.; Niacin .3 mg.	Calcium: 9 mg.
Vitamin C: 30 mg.	Iron: .2 mg.
Protein: .8 gm.	Phosphorus: 11 mg.
Calories: 51	

Reported health benefits: This fruit has been recommended for cases of loss of weight and vigor or loss of strength, poor vision, poor digestion, nervous exhaustion, and loss of reproductive faculties.

Preparation: This fruit is ideal for eating raw or it may be made into a salad or blended in a blender with other fruits and vegetables.

PLANTAIN

Botanical information: Fruit of the tropical perennial herb *musa paradisiaca.*

Nutritive values:

Vitamin B: Thiamine .06 mg.;	Fat: .4 gm.
Riboflavin .04 mg.; Niacin .6mg.	Carbohydrates: 31.2 gm.
Vitamin C: 14 mg.	Calcium: 7 mg.
Protein: 1.1 gm.	Iron: .7 mg.
Calories: 119	Phosphorus: 30 mg.

Reported health benefits: There are no reported medicinal benefits other than the nutrient value of this fruit.

Preparation: This fruit is often baked or roasted, and served with the main course as a potato substitute.

To prepare, wash plantains, leave in skins, and place on a baking sheet in a pre-heated oven (350 degrees). Bake thirty to forty minutes, or until easily pierced with a fork. Remove from oven, split the skins and season with salt and pepper, or if preferred, with butter and brown sugar.

To saute, melt enough butter to coat the bottom of a heavy skillet. Peel and slice plantains and arrange in skillet. Saute slowly until golden. The flavor is delicious as it is, or add a dash of sherry just before serving if you want something a little different.

PLUM

Botanical information: The plum is the edible fruit of trees of the genus *Prunus* and especially of the tree known as *Prunus domestica,* or garden plum.

Nutritive values:

Vitamin A: 350 I.U. per 100 gm.   Fat: .2 gm.
Vitamin B: Thiamine .06 mg.;   Carbohydrates: 20.4 gm.
   Riboflavin .04 mg.; Niacin .5 mg.   Calcium: 17 mg.
Vitamin C: 5 mg.   Iron: .5 mg.
Protein: .7 gm.   Phosphorus: 20 mg.
Calories: 50   Potassium: 100 mg.

Reported health benefits: The plum has been recommended for liver disorders, constipation, piles (hemorrhoids), poor digestion, abdominal gas, obesity, bronchitis, tumors and skin eruptions.

Preparation: Plums and prunes (dried plums) are known to contain oxalic acid, a substance of benefit to the body in its natural state. However, when the food in which oxalic acid exists is boiled, the acid destroys the calcium supply in the body. In view of this, both the plum and the prune should be eaten in the natural state, without any cooking whatsoever.

POMEGRANATE

Botanical information: Fruit of the tree *Punica granatum.*

Nutritive values:

Vitamin A: trace   Fat: .3 gm.
Vitamin B: Thiamine .03 mg.;   Carbohydrates: 16.4 gm.
   Riboflavin .03 mg.; Niacin .3 mg.   Calcium: 11 mg.
Vitamin C: 4 mg.   Iron: .7 mg.
Protein: .5 gm.   Phosphorus: 17 mg.
Calories: 63

Reported health benefits: Pomegranate has a very cleansing and cooling effect on the system. It is a good blood purifier, and beneficial for the expulsion of worms, especially tapeworms. It is also reported to be helpful in relieving liver congestion, arthritis and obesity.

Preparation: Because the seeds cling so tightly to the skin, it is usually easiest just to juice this fruit; however, the seeds can be sucked from the skin and the healthful benefits obtained.

The juice can be taken straight, but is usually best enjoyed added to either carrot or apple juice, creating a delicious and healthful beverage.

POTATO, SWEET

Botanical information: The sweet potato is an edible tuber of *Batatas batatas* of the family *Solanaceae*.

Nutritive values:

Vitamin A: 7,700 I.U. per 100 gm.	Fat: .7 gm.
Vitamin B: Thiamine .09 mg.;	Carbohydrates: 27.9 gm.
Riboflavin .05 mg.; Niacin .6 mg.	Calcium: 30 mg.
Vitamin C: 22 mg.	Iron: .7 mg.
Protein: 1.8 gm.	Phosphorus: 49 mg.
Calories: 123	Potassium: 300 mg.

Reported health benefits: The sweet potato is a fine food for individuals engaged in heavy muscular work, as the large quantities of vitamins and minerals contribute to the required body strength necessary for hard labor. It is an easily digestible food and is good for stomach ulcers and inflamed conditions of the colon. It is a good food for persons suffering from low blood pressure and from poor blood circulation. Persons suffering from hemorrhoids find this food to be good for them, and the sweet potato is helpful in cases of diarrhea.

Preparation: There are numerous ways of preparing the sweet potato. It can be baked, boiled, candied, casseroled, creamed, fried, grilled, hashed, mashed, stewed and stuffed.

Probably the most delicious sweet potato is the potato baked in its jacket. The potatoes are first washed and blemishes removed. They are then baked in a moderate oven of 350°F. until easily pierced with a fork, usually from thirty to forty minutes. After removal from the oven, the potato is slit and a large piece of butter may be inserted into the slit for additional flavor, although the potato without the butter is tasty enough for most individuals.

Another method of preparing sweet potatoes is to parboil them until the skins will slip off easily. (To parboil means to boil partially.) They may then be rolled in finely chopped pecans and placed in a well-greased baking dish. A light coating of honey may then be poured over the potatoes. The dish should then be covered and baking done in a moderate oven of 350°F. for thirty minutes.

A popular sweet potato dish is to cook them with the skins on after carefully washing them. They usually taste best when boiled in slightly salted water. They are cooked until tender for from twenty to thirty minutes. After being cooked, the jackets are removed and they are served piping hot.

POTATO, WHITE

Botanical information: The potato is the edible tuber of the plant *Solanum tuberosum* of the family *Solanaceae.*

Nutritive values:

Vitamin A: 20 I.U. per 100 gm.   Fat: .1 gm.
Vitamin B: Thiamine .11 mg.;   Carbohydrates: 19.1 gm.
   Riboflavin .04 mg.; Niacin 1.2   Calcium: 11 mg.
   mg.   Iron: .7 mg.
Vitamin C: 17 mg.   Phosphorus: 56 mg.
Protein: 2.0 gm.   Potassium: 500 mg.
Calories: 83

Reported health benefits: The common or white potato has acquired the name of Irish potato, as it has long been a staple food of Ireland. The baked potato is a good body-building food and is easily digested. Medicinal uses include application of a cold crushed potato for relief of burns and making a poultice of raw, crushed or scraped potatoes for sore eyes, boils, and inflammation of the skin and adjacent tissue (erysipelas). For inflammation along the course of a nerve, a hot poultice of raw or crushed potato is an excellent remedy.

Preparation: White potatoes are baked, boiled, fried, mashed, scalloped, stuffed and whipped. For baking, the potato is washed, allowed to dry or dried with a towel, and then baked in a hot oven of 425°F. for about one hour or until tender when pierced with a fork. Before serving, it is best to cut across the flat side of the potato with a sharp knife and to then sprinkle with paprika for flavoring. Butter is often used on each side of the potato for a tastier dish, although caution must be exercised to avoid excessive use of fattening foods.

The new potatoes, with thin skin coverings, are often boiled without removal of their skins and boiled until a fork can penetrate and be removed without difficulty. They may be sprinkled with paprika or finely chopped parsley for flavoring, with perhaps a butter coating.

To make stuffed potatoes, the baked potato is cut in half and the insides are scooped out. The insides are then mashed until softened and various seasonings and spices are added for flavoring, together with hot milk or hot cream, whatever the needs of the individual may be. One who is convalescing from an illness, for example, may perhaps not be worrying about his diet and he may require the most nourishing foods available. After treatment by mashing with the ingredients mentioned, the potato is returned to the shell, sprinkled with paprika, chopped parsley or grated cheese, and then served. The grated cheese may be melted and browned by placing the dish of potatoes under the broiler.

Scalloped potatoes are made by slicing the potatoes paper thin, placing them in the bottom of a buttered casserole and sprinkling with some whole wheat flour and butter. Sliced onions are then laid over the potatoes and another layer of potatoes is laid over the onions. Various herbs and spices are then sprinkled over the top and hot milk is added to the whole. Paprika is then sprinkled over the top and the casserole is baked in a moderate oven of 375°F. for an hour or longer until the potatoes are tender and the top is browned. Grated cheese may be sprinkled over the top before placing into oven.

PRUNES, DRIED

Botanical information: *Prunus domestica,* the dried fruit of any one of several varieties of the common plum.

Nutritive values:

Vitamin A: 1,890 I.U. per 100 gm.

Vitamin B: Thiamine .10 mg.; Riboflavin .16 mg.; Niacin 1.7 mg.

Vitamin C: 3 mg.

Fat: .6 gm.

Carbohydrates: 71 gm.

Calcium: 11 mg.

Iron: .7 mg.

Phosphorus: 85 mg.

Protein: 2.3 gm.   Potassium: 810 mg.
Calories: 268

Reported health benefits: Prunes are excellent for increasing one's vitality and improving the blood circulation. Individuals who are anemic will benefit from prunes, and the value of prunes for constipation is so well known as to hardly be worth mentioning. They are also known to be beneficial to persons suffering from hemorrhoids. Prune juice is an excellent remedy for a sore throat.

Preparation: Prunes should be allowed to soak overnight rather than stewed or boiled because of the oxalic acid content. Boiling of foods containing oxalic acid has a tendency to remove the calcium content from the body.

Prunes may be mixed into breads, cakes, cookies, fillings, ice cream, pies and puddings. They are delicious when added to other foods, or even combined with other foods into sandwiches.

A delicious prune pudding may be made by taking a cup of mashed prunes and mixing the prunes in a mixing bowl with two cups of graham cracker crumbs, one-half cup honey, a cup of chopped nuts, a cup of coconut, and one-half cup milk or cream. The mixture may then be eaten as is or poured into a refrigerator tray lined with heavy wax paper and frozen.

PUMPKIN

Botanical information: The pumpkin is the large, round yellow fruit of the plant *Cucurbita pepo,* a large trailing vine with heart-shaped leaves.

Nutritive values:

Vitamin A: 3,400 I.U. per 100 gm.   Fat: .2 gm.
Vitamin B: Thiamine .05 mg.;   Carbohydrates: 7.3 gm.
   Riboflavin .08 mg.; Niacin .6 mg.   Calcium: 21 mg.
Vitamin C: 8 mg.   Iron: .8 mg.
Protein: 1.2 gm.   Phosphorus: 44 mg.
Calories: 31   Potassium: 200 mg.

Reported health benefits: The pumpkin is valuable for cases of dropsy (abnormal accumulations of fluids in cavities of the body), infected or inflamed intestines, stomach ulcers and hemorrhoids. Pumpkin also raises blood pressure and thus helps the blood in carrying nourishment to various parts of the body.

Preparation: Most pumpkins are used for pies, although pumpkin cookies and pumpkin custard dishes are popular. A good pumpkin pie recipe is to take two-thirds cup of brown sugar and mix it with two eggs and one and two-thirds cup of milk. Two teaspoons of pumpkin pie spice may be added to the mix, together with one and one-half cups of mashed, cooked pumpkin. Baking is done in a very hot oven of 450°F. for ten minutes, followed with baking for thirty-five minutes or longer at a temperature of 325°F. or until a knife inserted in the center comes out clean. One-third cup of chopped nuts may be added to the mixture before baking.

Pumpkin cookies are made by taking one and one-half cups of cooked, mashed pumpkin and mixing with two eggs, two and one-half cups of whole wheat flour, four teaspoons of baking powder, one and one-quarter cups of brown sugar, and one-half cup of shortening, such as 100 per cent corn oil. Some spices, such as ginger, nutmeg, and cinnamon (one-half teaspoon each) should be added, and a cup of raisins, a cup of chopped nuts, and the juice of half a lemon to add to the taste of the final product. After all ingredients are well-blended, a teaspoon of the mixture at a time may be dropped onto a cookie sheet well lubricated with corn oil or other shortening. With the oven preheated to 400°F., baking for about fifteen minutes will suffice.

Two-thirds cup of mashed pumpkin may be sweetened with one-quarter cup of brown sugar and then mixed into the standard custard sauce, prepared by combining two eggs with one-quarter cup brown sugar, two cups of milk that have just been brought to a boil, one-half teaspoon of vanilla extract, and one-eighth teaspoon of salt. The custard sauce mix should be cooked in the top portion of a double boiler or simmered very slowly with constant stirring in a single boiler until the mixture is thick enough to coat a spoon when it is dipped into the mixture and removed.

PUMPKIN SEEDS

Botanical information: The seeds are from the pumpkin vine known as *Cucurbita pepo*.

Nutritive values:

Vitamin A: 70 I.U. per 100 gm.
Vitamin B: Thiamine .24 mg.; Riboflavin .19 mg.; Niacin 2.4 mg.

Fat: 46.7 gm.
Carbohydrates: 15.0 gm.
Calcium: 51 mg.

Iron: 11.2 mg.
Phosphorus: 1144 mg.

Protein: 29.0 gm.
Calories: 553

Reported health benefits: The pumpkin seed contains nutrients that have led it to be known as the building stone of the male hormone. Much relief from prostate problems has been obtained from this wonderful seed.

It is also recommended in cases of constipation, and a tea of the seeds is valuable for tape and other worm elimination.

Preparation: The best way to eat pumpkin seeds is just as they are; a handful of the raw or roasted hulled seeds are an excellent substitute for candy, providing many valuable nutrients that most snacks do not have. The seeds are also a good addition to a vegetable or fruit salad, and are often added to milk and fruit blender drinks, adding to its flavor and nutritive value.

QUINCE

Botanical information: Fruit of the *Cydonia cydonia* tree.

Nutritive values:

Vitamin A: 40 I.U. per 100 gm.
Vitamin B: Thiamine .02 mg.;
  Riboflavin .03 mg.; Niacin .2 mg.
Vitamin C: .5 mg.
Protein: .4 gm.
Calories: 57
Fat: .1 gm.
Carbohydrates: 15.3 gm.
Calcium: 11 mg.
Iron: .7 mg.
Phosphorus: 17 mg.

Reported health benefits: Beneficial in cases of sluggish liver, constipation, arthritis, and acidosis.

Preparation: This fruit should be eaten only when very ripe, or else it is very acid-forming. It should not be eaten raw, and is usually made into jellies, preserves or marmalades.

To make a quince honey jelly, wash, pare and core one and one-half pounds quinces. Add two and one-half cups water to parings and cook for thirty minutes. Grate or grind quinces or slice very thin. Weigh pulp and use one pound. Add two tablespoons lemon juice and strained liquid from parings. Cook until tender, add three cups sugar, and cook until syrup gives test for jelly. Pour into sterile glasses and seal with paraffin.

RADISH

Botanical information: The radish is the antiscorbutic root of the plant *Raphanus sativus,* commonly eaten raw as a salad or relish.

Nutritive values:

Vitamin A: 30 I.U. per 100 gm.
Vitamin B: Thiamine .03 mg.;
   Riboflavin .02 mg.; Niacin .3 mg.
Vitamin C: 24 mg.
Protein: 1.2 gm.
Calories: 20

Fat: .1 mg.
Carbohydrates: 4.2 gm.
Calcium: 37 mg.
Iron: 1.0 mg.
Phosphorus: 31 mg.
Potassium: 130 mg.

Reported health benefits: Radishes have been reported as beneficial for the teeth, gums, nerves, hair and nails. They are also said to stimulate the appetite and to relieve nervous exhaustion. In addition, reports indicate that radishes will relieve cases of constipation and catarrh, the condition of fluids running from mucous membranes. Additional reports reveal that this vegetable helps to reduce overweight or obesity and will dissolve gallstones. It is also claimed that radishes are helpful in cases of tuberculosis. Radishes also have a mild diuretic effect, increasing the production of urine by the kidneys.

Preparation: Radishes may be eaten raw or the juice extracted by the use of a juicer. They are often used after merely washing them and added to other items of a vegetable salad such as celery, lettuce and carrots.

A popular way of cooking radishes is to remove the leaves and root, wash them and place them in a pan. Add sufficient water to cover the radishes and cook uncovered for fifteen to twenty minutes. As in all cooking of vegetables, the water remaining after preparation usually has a large quantity of vitamins and minerals and makes a healthy drink, either alone or with herbs and spices added for a delicious herb tea to accompany the meal.

Braised radishes are prepared by slicing the washed radishes and cooking them in a covered pan for about ten minutes. The radishes are then removed from the pan and cooked in butter for five minutes, after which time one-half teaspoon of salt is added to one-quarter cup of milk or cream and the radishes allowed to simmer for five minutes or longer. This recipe calls for three bunches of radishes and will serve six to eight persons.

RAISINS

Botanical information: Raisins are dried grapes, usually of the variety containing much sugar and either sun-dried or oven-dried. The most common varieties are known as large or ordinary raisins, sultanas or seedless raisins, and currants or Corinth raisins.

Nutritive values:

Vitamin A: 50 I.U. per 100 gm.	Fat: .5 gm.
Vitamin B: Thiamine .15 mg.;	Carbohydrates: 71.2 gm.
Riboflavin .08 mg.; Niacin .5 mg.	Calcium: 78 mg.
Vitamin C: trace	Iron: 3.3 mg.
Protein: 2.3 gm.	Phosphorus: 129 mg.
Calories: 268	Potassium: 575 mg.

Reported health benefits: Raisins are considered a valuable strength-building food and are desirable for persons who are weak, emaciated or anemic. It will also help cases of tuberculosis, low blood pressure, constipation, and some cases of heart disease. The juice of soaked or stewed raisins has been found to be a good remedy for sore throats, asthma and cases of catarrh (mucus running from mucous membrane).

Preparation: Raisins are used in many ways. They are often used in bread, cookies, cakes, pies, puddings, sauces, stews and stuffings.

A delicious pudding is made by first rinsing about three-quarters cup of raisins and combining the raisins with one-half cup honey and four cups of whole wheat bread cubes. The mixture is cooked over a low heat for two or three minutes and stirred until the bread absorbs the honey. A quart of milk is then blended into the mixture, together with five eggs, one-quarter cup of brown sugar, one-quarter teaspoon salt, and two teaspoons of vanilla extract. The mixture is then poured into a buttered baking dish and sprinkled with nutmeg. The dish should then be placed in a pan of hot water and baked in a moderate oven of 350°F. for one hour, or until a knife inserted in the center comes out clean. This will serve six to eight persons.

RASPBERRIES, BLACK

Botanical information: The black raspberry is called *Rubus occidentalis,* while the red raspberry is named *Rubus idaeus.*

Nutritive values:

Vitamin B: Thiamine .02 mg.;	Fat: 1.6 gm.
Riboflavin .07 mg.; Niacin .3 mg.	Carbohydrates: 15.7 gm.
Vitamin C: 24 mg.	Calcium: 40 mg.
Protein: 1.5 gm.	Iron: .9 mg.
Calories: 74	Phosphorus: 37 mg.

Note: The red raspberry is similar in nutritive value to the black, except that in a quantity of 100 grams of the red there are 130 I.U. of Vitamin A.

Reported health benefits: Raspberries have been found to be valuable for destroying body worms, and they also have the effect of relieving menstrual cramps and removing excess fat of the body. They are also recommended for cases of constipation, high blood pressure and congested liver. The leaves of the raspberry bush are excellent for making a tea that is very effective for diarrhea. The tea should be allowed to cool before drinking it.

Preparation: To prepare a tea drink with raspberry leaves, use one ounce of the leaves. Pour one and one-half pints of water into a pan of leaves and simmer for twenty minutes. The warm tea helps in easing menstrual flow and helps to make childbirth easier when taken during pregnancy.

RHUBARB

Botanical information: This is a hardy perennial herb named *Rheum rhaponticum.*

Nutritive values:

Vitamin A: 30 I.U. per 100 gm.	Fat: .1 gm.
Vitamin B: Thiamine .01 mg.;	Carbohydrates: 3.8 gm.
Riboflavin none; Niacin .1 mg.	Calcium: 51 mg.
Vitamin C: 9 mg.	Iron: .5 mg.
Protein: .5 gm.	Phosphorus: 25 mg.
Calories: 16	Potassium: 510 mg.

Reported health benefits: Rhubarb has the effect of increasing the flow of saliva as well as gastric juice and bile. It also aids in peristalsis, the movement for elimination of the contents of the small and large intestines. Rhubarb contains high quantities of oxalic acid and should therefore be avoided by persons suffering from rheumatism or arthritis. It is recommended for cases of constipation, obesity, tumors, neuritis and bronchitis. It helps to remove worms from the body.

Preparation: Rhubarb is commonly used in cakes, jams, marmalade, pies, puddings, salads and sauces. A typical delightful rhubarb treat is to blend one-half cup butter with one-half cup of brown sugar. Add two eggs and beat well. Add one-half teaspoon of nutmeg, one-half teaspoon vanilla flavoring, two cups of toasted whole wheat bread cubes and two bananas, sliced. Half of the mixture is placed in a buttered baking pan and four cups of fresh diced rhubarb stems are placed over the mixture, sprinkled with another half-cup of brown sugar, and covered with the balance of the mixture. Baking is done in a moderate oven of 375°F. for about forty minutes, or until the rhubarb is tender.

RICE, BROWN

Botanical information: Rice is the grain or seed of the grass *Oryza sativa.* It is an aquatic plant widely cultivated in warm climates on wet land.

Nutritive values:

Vitamin B: Thiamine .32 mg.; Riboflavin .05 mg.; Niacin 4.6 mg.

Protein: 7.5 gm.

Calories: 360

Fat: 1.7 gm.

Carbohydrates: 77.7 gm.

Calcium: 39 mg.

Iron: 2 mg.

Phosphorus: 303 mg.

Potassium: 150 mg.

Reported health benefits: Brown rice is an easily digested starch food and provides all of the necessary carbohydrate requirements. In addition to the vitamins and minerals mentioned, this food contains Vitamin B_6 (pantothenic acid) and Vitamin K. It is a nourishing and body-building food, and is the principal food of the mass of the population of such Asiatic countries as China and India. It is reported as beneficial for stomach or intestinal ulcers and for the relief of diarrhea. Because of the mineral content, it is said to supply important nutrients for the hair, teeth, nails, muscles and bones.

Preparation: Rice can be prepared in a variety of interesting ways.

It is often prepared as a cereal, made into balls, cakes, cookies, custards, muffins, omelets, puddings, waffles, and many other preparations. Rice should not be overcooked, and the general rule should be observed that food should be cooked only enough for softening sufficiently for comfort in the chewing or masticating process.

A rice casserole can be prepared by lining a baking dish with hot cooked rice and then filling the center with any one of a number of foods. More rice is then used to cover the food, and the dish is placed in a hot oven of 425°F. for fifteen minutes or until browned.

For a delicious rice pudding serving six persons, take one-half cup brown rice and stir into a quart of milk together with one-half cup of brown sugar, one-half teaspoon of cinnamon or nutmeg (or both), and one-half teaspoon salt. Pour the mixture into a baking dish and bake for three hours in an oven of 275°F. Stir frequently during the first hour, and during the last half hour stir in one-half cup raisins and, if richness is desired, add two eggs to the mixture.

RUTABAGAS

Botanical information: A cultivated plant *(Brassica campestris rutabaga)* or its edible ovoid or globular yellowish root.

Nutritive values:

Vitamin A: 330 I.U. per 100 gm.	Fat: .1 gm.
Vitamin B: Thiamine .07 mg.;	Carbohydrates: 8.9 gm.
Riboflavin .08 mg.; Niacin .9 mg.	Calcium: 55 mg.
Vitamin C: 36 mg.	Iron: .4 mg.
Protein: 1.1 gm.	Phosphorus: 41 mg.
Calories: 38	Potassium: 170 mg.

Reported health benefits: This vegetable is considered good for cases of constipation and it will help to remove gas from the stomach. It has also been reported as helpful in the removal of intestinal worms.

Preparation: After cutting off the tail of the root and the tops, the bulb of the vegetable is cut into slices or cubes and boiled in a small amount of water in a covered pan from twenty to forty minutes, or until it is sufficiently softened to be edible. Rutabaga is often mixed with potatoes and other vegetables for variety in flavoring. Spices may also be added for extra flavor.

RYE

Botanical information: The grain or seed produced by the cereal grass *Secale cereale*.

Nutritive values:

Vitamin B: Thiamine .43 mg.;
Riboflavin .22 mg.; Niacin 1.6 mg.
Protein: 12.1 gm.
Calories: 334

Fat: 1.7 gm.
Carbohydrates: 73.4 gm.
Calcium: 38 mg.
Iron: 3.7 mg.
Phosphorus: 376 mg.

Reported health benefits: Rye is a good general body builder, aiding in muscle development, and is good for the glands.

Preparation: Whole rye can be ground into flour and used in the preparation of bread, pancakes and other baked goods, or the flour may be purchased already ground at most health food stores and some grocery stores.

To prepare whole or cracked rye, bring four and one-half to six cups of water to which one teaspoon salt has been added to a rapid boil over direct heat on top of double boiler. Gradually sprinkle in one and one-half cups cereal and boil gently three to five minutes, stirring occasionally. Cover and place over simmering water in lower part of double boiler. Cook for about three hours or until the grain is tender.

SALSIFY (OYSTER PLANT)

Botanical information: European biennial *Tragopogan porrifoluis*.
Nutritive values:

Vitamin A: 10 I.U. per 100 gm.
Vitamin B: Thiamine .04 mg.;
Riboflavin .04 mg.; Niacin .3 mg.
Vitamin C: 11 mg.
Protein: 2.9 gm.
Calories: 13 to 82

Fat: .6 gm.
Carbohydrates: 18 gm.
Calcium: 47 mg.
Iron: 1.5 mg.
Phosphorus: 66 mg.

Reported health benefits: Salsify or oyster plant, as it is sometimes known, is recommended as a good general body builder; also beneficial in cases of insomnia, colitis and neuritis.

Preparation: There are a number of delicious preparations of this vegetable. For the basic cooking take eight roots salsify; wash, scrape clean, and slice thin into water to which one tablespoon vinegar has been added. Drain. Cover with boiling water, add one teaspoon salt, and cook until tender, forty to fifty minutes. To serve, add butter and pepper.

To make mock oysters, combine two cups mashed cooked salsify, one egg, one-half teaspoon salt, a dash of paprika and one tablespoon butter. Shape into cakes and brown in fat.

For an easy and very tasty casserole, take three and one-half cups cooked salsify and place in alternate layers with three-quarters cup chopped celery. Add one cup sauce, made with milk, butter and flour, and cover with bread crumbs (about one-half cup) and dot with butter. Bake in moderate oven (375 degrees) for about twenty-five minutes.

SAPOTE

Botanical information: Fruit of the West Indian marmalade tree.

Nutritive values:

Vitamin A: 410 I.U. per 100 gm.   Fat: .6 gm.
Vitamin B: Thiamine .01 mg.;   Carbohydrates: 31.6 gm.
   Riboflavin .02 mg.; Niacin 1.8 mg.   Calcium: 39 mg.
Vitamin C: 20 mg.   Iron: 1.0 mg.
Protein: 1.8 gm.   Phosphorus: 28 mg.
Calories: 125

Reported health benefits: The sapote, or sapodilla as it is sometimes known, has no particular health benefits; however, it has many valuable nutrients and should be eaten when available for the vitamins and minerals.

Preparation: Wash, peel and slice fruit away from the seeds. Arrange on a dessert plate garnished with green leaves and a touch of other fruit for contrast (strawberries or apricots in season, or your choice).

Sapote, put through a sieve or blender, may be used in ices, sherbets or beverages. The creamy texture and subtle flavor takes them out of the ordinary.

SESAME SEEDS

Botanical information: *Sesamum indicum,* an East-Indian herb. Same as gama grass.

Nutritive values:

Vitamin A: 15 I.U. per 100 gm.
Vitamin B: Thiamine 1.07 mg.;
   Riboflavin .1 mg.; Niacin 2.7 mg.

Protein: 9 gm.
Calories: 280

Fat: 24 gm.
Carbohydrates: 10 gm.
Calcium: 580 mg.
Iron: 5.2 mg.
Phosphorus: 308 mg.
Potassium: 360 mg.

Reported health benefits: Helpful in cases of constipation and for ridding the body of pus formations. It is also useful in clearing away the milk-like crust that forms on the face and head of an infant, as well as various chronic diseases of the skin. It will also often relieve local swelling or tumors. The Vitamin E content strengthens the nerves and heart. It will often cure liver ailments. Ample portions of the seeds will increase body weight for cases of emaciation. The seeds have also been found to be valuable in the removal of worms from the intestinal tract.

Preparation: The oil of the sesame seeds may be used for cooking and for salad dressings. It is preferable to olive oil, being less expensive and having a very pleasant flavor. As with olive oil, it may be used externally for soothing and healing in cases of sunburn or other burns, or for minor eruptions of the skin or skin inflammations. It is also used as a hair dressing. Many people have found it helpful in the removal of wrinkles when used as a facial massage.

A popular use for sesame seeds is to sprinkle them over rolls and cookies just prior to baking. After baking, the flavor resembles toasted almonds. The seeds are marketed both hulled and unhulled. Apparently the best grade of unhulled seed is a variety from Turkey.

The seed can be creamed into a spread for bread that gives strength and nourishment.

SOURSOP

Botanical information: Fruit of the tropical tree *anona muricata,* grown in tropical America.

Nutritive values:

Vitamin A: 10 I.U. per 100 gm.   Fat: .3 gm.

Vitamin B: Thiamine .07 mg.;   Carbohydrates: 16.3 gm.
  Riboflavin .05 mg.; Niacin .9 mg. Calcium: 14 mg.
Vitamin C: 20 mg.   Iron: .6 mg.
Protein: 1.0 gm.   Phosphorous: 27 mg.
Calories: 65

Reported health benefits: This exotic tropical fruit contains a bit of almost all vitamins, minerals, carbohydrates and some fat, protein and calories; it can be regarded almost as a complete food. It would be an ideal diet for someone wishing to adopt a slimming diet for removal of obesity and the conditions usually accompanying obesity such as heart, liver and kidney ailments.

Preparation: This fruit may be eaten raw or mixed with other fruits and vegetables as a salad.

SOYBEANS

Botanical information: *Glycine hispida,* a small erect herb of the bean family.

Nutritive values:

Vitamin A: 110 I.U. per 100 gm.   Fat: 18.1 gm.
Vitamin B: Thiamine 1.07 mg.;   Carbohydrates: 34.8 gm.
  Riboflavin .31 mg.; Niacin 2.3   Calcium: trace
  mg.   Iron: 8.0 mg.
Vitamin C: trace   Phosphorus: 586 mg.
Protein: 34.9 gm.   Potassium: 540 mg.
Calories: 331

Reported health benefits: Food prepared from the soybean has long been valuable as an excellent food for diabetics. It is easily digested and is one of the most nourishing and body-building foods in the world. It is especially good for growing children for aid in growth and development. It has a high lecithin content and is therefore excellent for mental fatigue and for protection against cholesterol deposits. It is also reported as preventing pellagra, the disease marked by disturbances of the stomach and intestines, skin eruptions, and nervous symptoms such as melancholia. Because of the high content of linoleic and linolenic acids (unsaturated fatty acids), this food is conducive to a healthy skin and has corrected many cases of eczema. The pure pressed oil is used for skin conditions, as it contains the natural vitamins and lecithin. Soybeans have about twenty times more alkaline than milk.

Preparation: Soybeans should be cooked slowly so that they will be more digestible, and thereby also avoid losing valuable vitamins and minerals so often boiled away.

Soy flour is popular for making bread, biscuits, muffins, pancakes and waffles. For those interested in a good bread recipe with a generous portion of soybean flour, take two cups of milk, bring to boil and remove from heat. Take one package of active dry or one cake of compressed yeast and soften it in one-quarter cup of warm water, and allow to stand for five minutes. Pour the scalded milk over one-quarter cup of brown sugar and add two and one-half tablespoons of pure corn oil, sesame oil or butter. Add two teaspoons salt, or the salt may be omitted for persons on a salt-free diet.

Mix all of the foregoing ingredients except the yeast in a large mixing bowl, adding, while still warm, one cup of whole wheat flour. Then add the yeast to the mixture, beating well. Add one and one-half cups of soy flour, continuing to beat until smooth. Keep two additional cups of whole wheat flour at hand and continue to add enough flour until a soft dough results. Turn out on lightly floured surface and let stand for five minutes. Knead until it is smooth and elastic. Place dough in a greased bowl and turn the dough so that the greased surface is on top. Cover and allow to stand in a warm place until the dough rises to twice its size, which will take about an hour.

Remove the cover, punch the dough down to a smaller size, cover again and allow to stand until the dough again increases to almost double its size. Remove dough onto lightly floured surface and cut dough in half, and allow to rest for five to ten minutes. Shape the dough into two loaves to fit greased loaf pans. Cover and again allow to rise until about doubled in size for about one hour, then bake at 400°F. pre-heated oven for about fifty minutes.

For more richness and sweetness, add honey to the mixture at the start of the baking instructions; raisins, nuts, dates or figs may be added.

SPINACH

Botanical information: *Spinacia oleracea* of the goosefoot family.

Nutritive values:

Vitamin A: 9,420 I.U. per 100 gm.   Fat: .3 gm.

Vitamin B: Thiamine .11 mg.; Carbohydrates: 3.2 gm.
Riboflavin .20 mg.; Niacin .6 mg. Calcium: 81 mg.
Vitamin C: 59 mg. Iron: 3.0 mg.
Protein: 2.3 gm. Phosphorus: 55 mg.
Calories: 20 Potassium: 470 mg.

Reported health benefits: Spinach has been found valuable for anemia, constipation, neuritis, nerve exhaustion, tumors, insomnia, arthritis, obesity, high blood pressure, bronchitis, and dyspepsia (chronic indigestion). It has also helped ailments of the kidney, bladder and liver. Spinach is one of the foods with ample iron. In addition, spinach contains choline and inositol, the substances that help to prevent arteriosclerosis, or hardening of the arteries. (These substances are also found in Dandelions and in Beet Tops.)

Spinach is a good source of Vitamin K, which aids in the formation of the blood substance required for clotting of blood.

Preparation: Spinach is best eaten uncooked, as cooking yields the free oxalic acid found in spinach and has the effect of eliminating the calcium from the bloodstream.

SQUASH, SUMMER

Botanical information: *Cucurbita pepo.* Summer squashes are usually small and eaten only when green, the seeds being cooked in them.

Nutritive values:

Vitamin A: 260 I.U. per 100 gm. Fat: .1 gm.
Vitamin B: Thiamine .05 mg.; Carbohydrates: 3.9 gm.
Riboflavin .09 mg.; Niacin .8 mg. Calcium: 15 mg.
Vitamin C: 17 mg. Iron: .4 mg.
Protein: .6 mg. Phosphorus: 15 mg.
Calories: 16 Potassium: 480 mg.

Reported health benefits: Summer and Zucchini squash have been found valuable for cases of high blood pressure, obesity, constipation, and for bladder and kidney disorders; summer squash is an exceptionally good food for hot climates.

Preparation: A good food for hot summer days is to take about two pounds of summer squash and steam them without adding water, cooking them until soft but firm in a steamer. The insides are then scooped out and mixed with about one-half cup chopped celery and a cup of cottage cheese. Place some walnut and pecan nut meats in the squash shells and fill over with the mixed filling, sprinkling cinnamon over the top. Place in pan, heat in oven briefly and serve.

SQUASH, WINTER

Botanical information: *Cucurbita maxima.* At least sixty varieties of winter and summer squashes are recognized by horticulturists.

Nutritive values:

Vitamin A: 4,950 I.U. per 100 gm.   Fat: .3 gm.
Vitamin B: Thiamine .05 mg.;   Carbohydrates: 8.8 gm.
    Riboflavin .12 mg.; Niacin .5 mg.   Calcium: 19 mg.
Vitamin C: 8 mg.   Iron: .6 mg.
Protein: 1.5 gm.   Phosphorus: 28 mg.
Calories: 38   Potassium: 510 mg.

Reported health benefits: The winter squash (Hubbard and Banana varieties) have more carbohydrates, vitamins, minerals and protein than the summer squash. This variety of squash is useful in cases of diarrhea, hemorrhoids, inflammation of the colon (colitis), and ulcerations of the stomach or intestines.

Experiments conducted in a Cleveland clinic demonstrated that foods containing high quantities of Vitamin A would dissolve kidney, bladder and gallstones, as well as prevent stones from forming. Winter squash is high in Vitamin A content and would therefore be considered valuable for this purpose.

A rough or dry condition of the skin is often due to a deficiency of Vitamin A, and winter squash will tend to make the skin healthy, smooth and firm. Case histories indicate that foods with high Vitamin A content will also improve the eyesight and even make hair grow.

Preparation: In cooking squash, it must be remembered, as with other vegetables, that steam-cooking (using the water within the squash itself) is the preferred method. Also, the squash should be cooked only long enough for softening.

A popular recipe is to take about four cups of raw squash and place into a steamer with one-quarter teaspoon of rosemary and one-quarter teaspoon of basil. Portions of other vegetables may be added, such as chopped carrots, celery or onions. Cook until soft but firm.

A delicious squash dessert may be made for six persons by

blending together three cups of cooked and strained squash with two eggs, four tablespoons honey, two tablespoons lemon juice, four tablespoons of soy flour, two tablespoons of nutritional yeast, one-quarter teaspoon ground ginger, one-quarter teaspoon ground cinnamon, and one-quarter teaspoon ground nutmeg. After the mixture has been mixed until smooth, it should be poured into custard cups slightly oiled with peanut oil or other pure vegetable oil and baked at 350° for about thirty minutes. It may then be served hot or cold. For an extra fancy touch, the custard may be topped with yogurt.

SQUASH SEEDS

Botanical information: The seed of any one of the trailing annuals of the genus *Cucurbita.*

Nutritive values: The squash seed has the same nutritive value as the pumpkin seed.

Reported health benefits: Same as the pumpkin seed.

Preparation: The seed should be eaten raw and unsalted, either by the handful as snacks or added to fruit and vegetable salads for added nutrition. Squash seeds may also be ground in a nut chopper and added to blender drinks.

STRAWBERRY

Botanical information: The fruit of the plant of the genus *Fragaria.* Technically, the real fruit is the seed-like *achene* on the surface.

Nutritive values:

Vitamin A: 60 I.U. per 100 gm.
Vitamin B: Thiamine .03 mg.;
  Riboflavin .07 mg.; Niacin .3 mg.
Vitamin C: 60 mg.
Protein: .8 gm.
Calories: 37
Fat: .5 mg.
Carbohydrates: 8.3 gm.
Calcium: 28 mg.
Iron: .8 mg.
Phosphorus: 27 mg.
Potassium: 220 mg.

Reported health benefits: This is highly rated as a skin-cleansing food, even though skin eruptions may appear at first in some cases. It is also known to clean or rid the blood of harmful toxins. Strawberries have been recommended for a sluggish liver, gout, rheumatism, constipation, high blood pressure, catarrh and skin cancer. It has also been reported to help cases of syphilis. Crushed strawberries can be made into a poultice and applied to relieve sore eyes and cases of ringworm. Equal portions of strawberry leaves, parsley and blueberry leaves may be mixed together for a kidney remedy, as well as for diabetes. Pour some hot water over a teaspoonful of the dried and powdered leaf mixture and allow to steep for about ten minutes. The drink should be taken four times a day, spaced from morning until·bedtime.

The strawberry, when cut in half and rubbed on the teeth and gums, is said to remove tartar from the teeth and strengthen and heal the gums. The juice should be allowed to remain on the teeth as long as possible in order to dissolve the tartar. The mouth may then be rinsed with warm water.

Preparation: Strawberries are basically a dessert and are usually served at the end of the meal. However, there are ways of including the strawberries as a part of the main dish. For example, they may be included in an egg omelet by mashing the strawberries and mixing with eggs, the quantity depending upon the number of persons to be served. For more nutrition, unsweetened fruit juices may be added, and for flavoring add the grated rind of one-half orange and one-quarter teaspoon of crushed anise seeds.

A healthy, nutritious and delicious drink may be prepared by mixing two cups of fresh strawberries with two cups of milk, adding three tablespoons of honey for additional sweetening. This will serve from four to six persons.

Perhaps the simplest method of serving strawberries is to wash them after removal of the stems and serve on small dishes with a light application of honey.

SUNFLOWER SEEDS

Botanical information: These seeds are of the plant of the genus *Helianthus.*

Nutritive values:

Vitamin A: 50 I.U. per 100 gm.

Vitamin B: Thiamine 1.96 mg.; Riboflavin .23 mg.; Niacin 5.4 mg.

Fat: 47.3 gm.

Carbohydrates: 19.9 gm.

Calcium: 120 mg.

Iron: 47.3 mg.

Phosphorus: 6 mg.

Protein: 24.0 gm.

Calories: 560

Reported health benefits: This seed is one of the best natural foods and should be included in everyone's diet. It nourishes the entire body, supplying it with many vital elements needed for growth and repair. This seed is good for weak eyes, poor fingernails, tooth decay, arthritis, and dryness of skin. The oil is soothing to the skin and a good hair dressing.

Preparation: This seed should always be eaten raw, either by the handful or as an addition to fruit and vegetable salads.

Sunflower seeds are also sold as flour, meal and butter—equally nutritious, and useful for many purposes in menu planning.

A delicious beverage is made by taking one cup of sunflower seeds and blending until well chopped; add two cups of water or fruit juice and liquefy until well mixed. Honey and banana can be added to this for nutrients and flavor.

TAMARIND

Botanical information: Fruit of the tree *Tamarindus Indica.*

Nutritive values:

Vitamin A: 30 I.U. per 100 gm.
Vitamin B: Thiamine .34 mg.; Riboflavin .14 mg.; Niacin 1.2 mg.
Vitamin C: 2 mg.
Proteins: 2.8 gm.
Calories: 239
Fat: .6 gm.
Carbohydrates: 62.5 gm.
Calcium: 74 mg.
Iron: 2.8 mg.
Phosphorus: 113 mg.

Reported health benefits: A cooling medicinal drink can be made of this fruit that is beneficial in fevers; make an infusion by taking one ounce of pulp, pour one quart of boiling water over this, and allow to steep for one hour. Strain and drink tepid. Drink this slowly, one-half diluted every two to three hours. Tamarind is an excellent laxative and is used as a diuretic remedy for bilious disorders, jaundice, and catarrh.

Preparation: Tamarind is made into a cooling beverage. It is used for preserving fish and, pressed into sugar or syrup, it is preserved as a fruit.

TANGELO

Botanical information: A loose-skinned orange-like fruit. It is a hybrid between the common tangerine and the grapefruit.

Nutritive values:

Fat: .1 gm.
Carbohydrates: 9.7 gm.

Vitamin C: 27 mg.
Protein: .5 gm.
Calories: 41

Reported health benefits: Tangelos have most of the same health benefits as tangerines, although they do not have the vitamin and mineral content of the tangerine.

Preparation: The most common use of the tangelo is to peel it and eat it from the hand, or it may be added to a fruit salad or made into juice.

TANGERINE

Botanical information: The tangerine is a small red-skinned orange.

Nutritive values:

Vitamin A: 420 I.U. per 100 gm.
Vitamin B: Thiamine .07 mg.;
   Riboflavin .03 mg.; Niacin .2 mg.
Vitamin C: 31 mg.
Protein: .8 gm.
Calories: 44

Fat: .3 gm.
Carbohydrates: 10.9 gm.
Calcium: 33 mg.
Iron: .4 mg.
Phosphorus: 23 mg.
Potassium: 110 mg.

Reported health benefits: Tangerines have been recommended for obesity, bronchitis, pneumonia, rheumatism, arthritis, asthma, catarrh, diabetes, high blood pressure, and various skin ailments. They have also been recommended for reducing fevers and for relieving conditions of congestion of the liver. There are also reports that tangerines are valuable for syphilis.

Preparation: The most common use of the tangerine is to peel it and serve it on a plate as a dessert, or to mix it with other fruits or berries.

TAPIOCA

Botanical information: Genus: *Manihot,* of the *spurge* family. The plant (herb) is also known as Cassava. Juice pressed from the root is heated on plates or dried in the sun and becomes tapioca.

Nutritive values:

Tapioca does not contain Vitamins A, B or C.

Protein: .6 gm.

Calories: 360

Fat: .2 gm.

Carbohydrates: 86.4 gm.

Calcium: 12 mg.

Iron: 1 mg.

Phosphorus: 12 mg.

Reported health benefits: Studies indicate that tapioca is valuable for stomach ulcers, as well as ulcers of the intestines. It has also been found beneficial for inflamed conditions of the colon as well as for diarrhea. It is valued as a light nutritious food for invalids.

Preparation: To prepare a tapioca omelet, add two tablespoons of quick-cooking tapioca to three-quarters cup of milk that has just been scalded, that is, brought to a boil but quickly taken off the heat. Spices may be added for flavoring and after thorough mixing, place in double boiler or cook over simmering heat for twenty minutes. A tablespoon of butter may then be added with four egg yolks that have first been beaten well. The four egg whites should then be stiffly beaten and folded into the mixture, after which the batter should be poured into a hot buttered skillet and baked in a moderate oven of 350°F. for twenty minutes. This will serve four persons.

A delicious tapioca pudding dessert may be made by first beating four egg whites. A rounded tablespoon of gelatine is dissolved into one-half cup of boiling water and stirred vigorously, after which one-half cup of cold water is added to the mix. When the mix is cool, add it slowly to the egg whites and add one-half cup of honey and two tablespoons of tapioca powder. Stir until the mixture becomes firm and serve. If desired, it may be cooled in the refrigerator before serving. Some of the whipped egg whites or some yogurt may be used as a topping.

TOMATO

Botanical information: A fruit technically, but generally accepted as a vegetable, the plant is known as *Lycopersicon* of the family *Solanaceae*.

Nutritive values:

Vitamin A: 1,100 I.U. per 100 gm.

Vitamin B: Thiamine .06 mg.;

Fat: .3 gm.

Carbohydrates: 4 gm.

Riboflavin .04 mg.; Niacin .05 mg.

Calcium: 11 mg.

Vitamin C: 23 mg.

Iron: .6 mg.

Vitamin K: Amount uncertain.

Phosphorus: 27 mg.

Protein: 1.0 gm.

Potassium: 360 mg.

Calories: 20

Reported health benefits: The tomato is a natural antiseptic and protects against infection. Ample consumption of tomatoes is reported to improve the skin and purify the blood. It is also said to help cases of gout, rheumatism, tuberculosis, high blood pressure and sinus trouble. It has been indicated for cases of congestion of the liver as well as for dissolving of gallstones. It is also reported to relieve gas in the stomach, as well as colds and obesity. In addition, it is reported to help in the removal of pimples from the skin, and when applied externally as a poultice or when eaten is reported to relieve cases of ringworm. The nicotinic acid in tomatoes helps to reduce cholesterol in the blood, while the Vitamin K in tomatoes helps to prevent hemorrhages.

Preparation: There are innumerable ways of preparing tomatoes, but the most popular and healthiest is to simply slice them and eat them as they are in their natural state. Of course, with tomatoes, as with other plants, there is a considerable difference between plants grown in rich, organic soil without pesticides and plants grown in depleted soil heavily saturated with poisons for destruction of insects. Every effort should be made to obtain the rich and nourishing plants grown organically. Not only is there a great difference in the taste, but the nutritive values also vary.

Tomatoes can be baked, broiled, canned, scrambled with eggs, served as side dishes, mixed with other vegetables as a salad, made into a sandwich with lettuce or with other foods, stewed, made into soups and stuffed with beans, spinach or other vegetables.

Tomatoes are baked by cutting off the tops and removing the pulp, mixing the pulp with chopped green pepper or other vegetables such as chopped carrots or cooked corn. Some herb spices may be added to the mixture, after which the tomato shells are filled and baked in a moderate oven of 375°F. for about twenty-five minutes.

Stewed tomatoes are prepared by peeling and cutting the tomatoes into pieces. The tomatoes are sprinkled with spices, placed in a saucepan, covered tightly to prevent escape of steam, and cooked slowly over a slow fire for about fifteen minutes, stirring occasionally. Onions may be added to the tomatoes for additional taste and flavoring.

To broil tomatoes, simply cut in half, sprinkle with herbs or spices, and place into oven. Usually, ten minutes with medium heat is sufficient for the tomatoes to become tender. Garnishing with parsley will add to the decorative effect, and of course the parsley is good to eat.

A delicious puffy omelet with tomatoes may be made by first beating egg whites until stiff, then beating the yolks until thick and lemon-colored. Use one tablespoon of hot water for each egg in the recipe and beat the hot water into the egg yolks. The yolks and whites are then folded together. Some peanut oil or butter is then placed into the omelet pan and the egg mixture allowed to cook over low heat until it is puffy and light brown underneath. The pan is then placed in a moderate oven of 350°F. for ten to fifteen minutes or until the top is dry. Cut across the center of the omelet and spread several slices of tomatoes, cut thin, over one half of the omelet, and use a spatula to lift the other half and cover the tomatoes, then serve.

A delicious and nourishing cream of tomato soup is made by adding two cups of cooked tomatoes (cooked for fifteen minutes with a tablespoon of chopped onion, a dash of cayenne pepper and some mixed spices) to a quart of milk barely brought to a boil, adding the milk gradually and stirring constantly. A tablespoon of honey may be added for sweetening.

TURNIP

Botanical information: *Brassica campestris.* The yellow turnip is called the rutabaga.

Nutritive values:

Vitamin A: trace

Vitamin B: Thiamine .05 mg.; Riboflavin .07 mg.; Niacin .5 mg.

Vitamin C: 28 mg.

Protein: 1.1 gm.

Calories: 32

Fat: .2 gm.

Carbohydrates: 7.1 gm.

Calcium: 40 mg.

Iron: .5 mg.

Phosphorus: 34 mg.

Potassium: 345 mg.

Reported health benefits: The turnip roots are considered valuable for constipation and for tuberculosis. They also are reported to relieve nervousness and insomnia and are reputed to be good for the teeth and gums when eaten raw, tending to clean the teeth. Some honey added to the water from the boiling of turnip roots is reported to relieve coughs, throat hoarseness and asthma.

Preparation: Turnip roots are excellent for salads, as they can be readily chewed. However, if the soft turnip is desired, boil in a small amount of water for approximately twenty minutes, after first scrubbing off the soil and cutting into slices or cubes. Sprinkle with spices or herbs when serving.

A popular method of baking turnips is to cut them into cubes and place them into a baking dish with a little water and honey. Some vegetable oil may be poured sparingly into the pan, just enough to prevent the turnips from sticking to the pan.

A delicious and nourishing turnip soup can be made by adding two tablespoons of chopped onion to three cups of water or milk (or part water and part milk) together with two cups of mashed turnips and one cup of mashed potatoes. The soup is cooked on low heat for about twenty minutes and served with chopped parsley and a dash of paprika. Other spices may be added for additional flavoring.

TURNIP GREENS

Botanical information: *Brassica Campestris.*

Nutritive values:

Vitamin A: 9,540 I.U. per 100 gm.
Vitamin B: Thiamine .09 mg.; Riboflavin .46 mg.; Niacin .8 mg.
Vitamin C: 136 mg.
Vitamin E: amount undetermined.
Vitamin K: amount undetermined.
Protein: 2.9 gm.
Calories: 30

Fat: .4 gm.
Carbohydrates: 5.4 gm.
Calcium: 259 mg.
Iron: 2.4 mg.
Phosphorus: 50 mg.

Reported health benefits: Because of the richness of turnip top greens in vitamins and minerals, they are considered excellent for persons suffering from anemia, poor appetite, tuberculosis, obesity, high blood pressure, bronchitis, asthma, liver ailments, gout, and bladder disorders. In addition, turnip greens are reputed to help the complexion, purify the blood, reduce acidity, and destroy bacterial toxins in the bloodstream (toxemia).

Preparation: Turnip greens may be prepared as a cooked vegetable, steaming them for twenty to thirty minutes after they have been cleaned and cut into small pieces. They should be prepared in the smallest amount of water; if a steam cooker is available, this should be used to steam-cook without any water whatsoever. The high content of potassium and calcium in turnip greens makes this vegetable especially suitable for young and old alike.

WALNUTS

Botanical information: The walnut is the nut of any tree of the genus *Juglans.*

Nutritive values:

Vitamin A: 30 I.U. per 100 gm.

Vitamin B: Thiamine .48 mg.; Riboflavin .13 mg.; Niacin 1.2 mg.

Vitamin C: 3 mg.

Protein: 15.0 gm.

Calories: 654

Fat: 64.4 gm.

Carbohydrates: 15.6 gm.

Calcium: 83 mg.

Iron: 2.1 mg.

Phosphorus: 380 mg.

Potassium: 225 mg.

Reported health benefits: Walnuts are good for constipation, having a definite laxative effect. The many vitamins and minerals make this nut an excellent means for body and muscle building. It is known to benefit the teeth and gums. It improves the body's metabolism. Walnuts have been especially recommended for patients with liver ailments.

Preparation: Walnuts are used in puddings, pies, cakes, cookies, bread, and as fillings and stuffings. Of course, they may also be eaten alone as a delicious food or confection treat.

A delicious pudding is made with the help of the sweet potato. Take a pound of grated, uncooked sweet potatoes and mix with one-half cup of black walnut meats, adding one-half cup honey, three well-beaten eggs, two tablespoons melted butter, two cups milk, one teaspoon cinnamon, one-half teaspoon nutmeg, one-half teaspoon allspice, and one-half cup raisins. After mixing all ingredients, the batter is poured into a buttered baking dish and baked in a slow oven of 325°F. for one hour, stirring occasionally. This will serve six persons.

A popular food for children is to prepare a walnut filling for cookies. A healthy cookie dough is prepared by using three and one-half cups of whole wheat flour, one cup of honey, three-quarters cup of vegetable or peanut oil, two well-beaten eggs, three teaspoons of baking powder, one-third cup milk, and one-half teaspoon vanilla flavoring. First, the oil and honey are mixed together and the eggs added. The dry ingredients are then mixed together and added alternately with the milk and the vanilla, mixing well after each addition. The dough is rolled out one-eighth inch thick on a floured pastry cloth. Pieces are cut out with a cookie cutter and a filling of chopped walnuts mixed with honey, whole wheat flour and some lemon juice, and sufficient water to make a jelly-like filling is placed in the center of the cookie dough. Another piece of dough is used to cover the filling, thereafter pinching the edges together. The filled cookies may then be topped with egg white and baked in a hot oven of 400°F. for fifteen minutes.

WATER CHESTNUTS

Botanical information: Water chestnut is the fruit of the aquatic plant, *Trapa Natans.*

Nutritive values:

Vitamin B: Thiamine .14 mg.; Riboflavin .20 mg.; Niacin 1.0 mg.
Vitamin C: 4 mg.
Protein: 1.4 gm.
Calories:: 27

Fat: .2 gm.
Carbohydrates: 19.0 gm.
Calcium: 4 mg.
Iron: .6 mg.
Phosphorus: 65 mg.

Reported health benefits: Water chestnuts are reported to be beneficial in cases of constipation, gas, worms, and intestinal putre-faction.

Preparation: Water chestnuts can be obtained at many large grocery stores or imported food stores. They may be added to salads but their more common appearance is with sauteed vegetables, Chinese style.

To make delicious vegetables using the Chinese method of cooking, which not only retains the natural flavor of the vegetables but also most of the nutrients, take one cup onions that have been sliced thin, one cup chopped green peppers, one cup chopped celery and tops, and one-half cup sliced mushrooms; saute briefly in one-quarter cup oil, remove from heat, and add one cup bean sprouts and one-half cup thinly sliced water chestnuts.

WATERCRESS

Botanical information: American watercress is *Cardamine rotundifolia;* English watercress is *Nasturtium officinale.*

Nutritive values:

Vitamin A: 4,720 I.U. per 100 gm.

Vitamin B: Thiamine .08 mg.;
Riboflavin .16 mg.; Niacin .8 mg.

Vitamin C: 77 mg.

Watercress also contains Vitamins E and G.

Protein: 1.7 gm.

Calories: 18

Fat: .3 gm.

Carbohydrates: 3.3 gm.

Calcium: 195 mg.

Iron: 2 mg.

Phosphorus: 46 mg.

Reported health benefits: Watercress has been recommended for eye disorders, excess weight, bleeding gums, arthritis, rheumatism, and hardening of the arteries (atherosclerosis). It has a high Vitamin C content (containing three times as much as lettuce). It has been highly recommended for kidney and liver disorders, and also for the relief of swelling in various body cavities (dropsy).

Preparation: There is no better way of using watercress than as a salad. It can either be used as a garnish or chopped up fine as an ingredient.

An eggplant and watercress salad is made by taking one small eggplant, which you skin and chop into small cubes. Salt well and leave for about an hour. Dry off the salt and marinate the eggplant in vinegar for about three hours. Dry and place in a salad bowl. Add one bunch watercress, one tablespoon chopped Spanish onion, one sliced tomato, one-quarter pound black olives, two hard boiled eggs, quartered, one teaspoon fresh chopped basil, and one teaspoon fresh parsley. Mix this well and add a vinegar dressing. Toss and serve.

A quick and simple cold soup is made by taking two cans chicken stock, two bunches watercress with the stalks cut off, juice of half a lemon, one tablespoon chopped onion, one cup yogurt, one-half cup heavy cream and some salt and pepper, placing these ingredients into the blender and blending until smooth. Refrigerate the soup until ready to serve. Garnish with pieces of watercress, some extra cream, and a paper-thin slice of lemon.

Watercress spread can be used as a dip for raw vegetables or on open-faced sandwiches. Remove the tougher stalks from one bunch of watercress. Place the watercress, one-half cup coarsely diced radishes, one cucumber, juice of one lemon, one-quarter cup sour cream, and some salt and pepper into the blender. Blend until smooth and refrigerate until ready to use.

WATERMELON

Botanical information: Watermelon is the large edible fruit of a trailing plant, *Citrullus,* of the gourd family.

Nutritive values:

Vitamin A: 590 I.U. per 100 gm.

Vitamin B: Thiamine .05 mg.; Riboflavin .05 mg.; Niacin .2 mg.

Vitamin C: 6 mg.

Protein: .5 gm.

Calories: 28

Fat: .2 gm.

Carbohydrates: 6.9 gm.

Calcium: 7 mg.

Iron: .2 mg.

Phosphorus: 12 mg.

Potassium: 600 mg.

Reported health benefits: Watermelon has been reported as very helpful in correcting abnormal kidney conditions. Apparently there is an ingredient in the seeds, Cucurbocitrin, which has the effect of dilating the capillaries, the tiny blood vessels of the body. Consequently, the pressure upon the large blood vessels is reduced.

Preparation: Watermelon wedges are popular as desserts and they are also used in fruit salads, pieces of watermelon being mixed with pieces of cantaloupes, pears, apples, and other fruits and berries.

For medicinal purposes, watermelon seed tea is prepared by crushing two teaspoons of the dried seeds and steeping them in a cup of hot water for an hour. Stir and strain. Drink a cup of this tea four times a day.

WHEAT

Botanical information: A grain, the edible product of a cereal grass *triticum sativum,* of several types: durim, hard spring, hard winter and soft winter.

Nutritive values:

Since the nutritive values of the various types of wheat are similar, only the values of the durim wheat are given.

Fat: 2.5 gm.

Vitamin B: Thiamine .66 mg.; Carbohydrates: 70.1 gm.

Riboflavin .12 mg.; Niacin 4.4 mg.

Calcium: 37 mg.
Iron: 4.3 mg.
Phosphorus: 346 mg.

Protein: 12.7 gm.
Calories: 332

Reported health benefits: Wheat is an excellent source of the B-Complex vitamins, and so it is a valuable addition to the diet. Besides the health properties derived from the B vitamins, it also is recommended in cases of arthritis, rheumatic fever, and perhaps in some types of cancer.

Preparation: Whole wheat flour is the perfect baking flour. Containing all the nutrients of the wheat, it is not only very healthful, but also adds delicious flavor to bread, pancakes, pastry, and all baked goods. It may be purchased at most stores in flour form; however, for the most nutrients and added flavor, it is best to buy whole wheat grain and grind it yourself.

Wheat may also be cooked like rice and served either plain or with a sauce, or it may be used as a base for casserole food preparations.

PART III
THE SYMPTOMATIC
LOCATOR INDEX

Anemia *(cont.)*

Symptom or Reference	*Food*	*Page*
	CHARD	83
	CHERRIES	84
	COLLARD GREENS	89
	CORN	89
	CURRANTS	93
	DANDELION GREENS	94
	DATES	95
	ENDIVES	98
	FIGS	99
	GRAPEFRUIT	104
	GUAVA	105
	HORSERADISH	107
	KALE	109
	KELP	110
	LEMONS	112
	LETTUCE	117
	MACADAMIA NUTS	120
	MUSTARD GREENS	124
	ORANGES	128
	PARSLEY	130
	PEACHES	132
	PEANUTS	133
	PEAS	134
	PECANS	135
	PEPPER	136
	PILINUTS	138
	PRUNES	145
	RAISINS	150
	SPINACH	158
	SOYBEANS	157
	TOMATOES	165
	TURNIP GREENS	168
	WATERCRESS	171
Anemia, cause of		48
Angina pectoris		16
Appetite, diminished	APRICOTS	62
	ASPARAGUS	63
	BEANS	67
	BEET GREENS	70
	BROCCOLI	73
	CABBAGE	75
	CANTALOUPE	76
	CARROTS	78
	CORN	89
	DANDELION GREENS	94
	ENDIVES	98
	KALE	109
	LETTUCE	117
	MUSTARD GREENS	124
	ORANGES	128
	PAPAYAS	130
	PARSLEY	130
	PEACHES	132
	PEAS	134
	PECANS	135
	POTATOES, SWEET	143
	PRUNES	145

Catarrh *(cont.)*

Symptom or Reference	*Food*	*Page*
	BLACKBERRIES	71
	BRUSSELS SPROUTS	74
	CARROTS	78
	CELERY	82
	CHARD	83
	CHERRIES	84
	ELDERBERRIES	98
	ENDIVES	98
	FIGS	99
	GARLIC	101
	GOOSEBERRIES	102
	GRAPEFRUIT	104
	GUAVA	105
	JERUSALEM ARTICHOKE	108
	KUMQUATS	112
	LETTUCE	117
	PARSLEY	130
	PEARS	133
	PINEAPPLE	139
	RADISHES	149
	RAISINS	150
	STRAWBERRIES	161
	TAMARINDS	163
	TANGERINES	164
Cellulose, value of		18
Cereals, whole grain		28
Chlorine		29
Cholesterol, cause of		26, 27, 28
Cholesterol, excessive	CORN	89
	OLIVES	126
	PEANUTS	133
	PEAS	134
	TOMATOES	165
Choline		54
Circulation, poor	DANDELION GREENS	94
	FIGS	99
	GUAVA	105
Cobalt		48
Colds	CARROTS	78
	BROCCOLI	73
	BRUSSELS SPROUTS	74
	CAULIFLOWER	81
	COLLARDS	89
	CURRANTS	93
	DANDELION GREENS	94
	ELDERBERRIES	98
	GARLIC	101
	GRAPEFRUIT	104
	GUAVA	105
	HORSERADISH	107
	KALE	109
	LEMONS	112
	ONIONS	127
	ORANGES	128
	PARSLEY	130
	PEPPERS	136
	SPINACH	158

Constipation *(cont.)*

Fever *(cont.)*

Indigestion *(cont.)*

Symptom or Reference	Food	Page
	SPINACH	158
	STRAWBERRIES	161
	TOMATOES	166
	TURNIPS	167
Indigestion, cause of		22
Infections, helpful for	BROCCOLI	73
	BRUSSELS SPROUTS	74
	CAULIFLOWER	81
	COLLARD GREENS	89
	CURRANTS	93
	ENDIVES	98
	GRAPEFRUIT	104
	GUAVA	105
	HORSERADISH	107
	KALE	110
	LEMONS	112
	ORANGES	128
	PARSLEY	130
	PEPPERS	136
	SPINACH	158
	TOMATOES	166
	TURNIPS	167
	WATERCRESS	171
Influenza, help for	LEEKS	112
	LEMONS	112
	ONIONS	127
Insect bites	LEMONS	112
Insomnia, help for	APPLES	60
	AVOCADO	64
	BARLEY	66
	BLACK WALNUTS	169
	BRAZIL NUTS	72
	CABBAGE	75
	CARROTS	78
	CELERY	82
	COLLARD GREENS	89
	CORN	89
	KALE	109
	LEEKS	112
	LETTUCE	117
	MUSHROOMS	123
	ONIONS	127
	PARSNIPS	131
	PECANS	135
	PEANUTS	133
	PEAS	134
	POTATOES	144
	RICE	152
	SALSIFY	154
	SOYBEANS	157
	SPINACH	158
	TOMATOES	166
	TURNIP GREENS	168
Inositol, need for		119
Insulin		22
Intestines, cleanser of	CABBAGE	75
	HAW	105

Thin *(cont.)*

Symptom or Reference	Food	Page
	CARROTS	78
	COCONUTS	87
	COLLARDS	89
	DANDELIONS	94
	GRAPEFRUIT	104
	LEMONS	112
	LETTUCE	117
	PEANUTS	133
	PRUNES	145
	TURNIPS	167
	WATERCRESS	171
Tongue, granulated	APPLES	60
	BEETS	69
	BLUEBERRIES	71
	BROCCOLI	73
	CABBAGE	75
	CARROTS	78
	COCONUTS	87
	COLLARD GREENS	89
	DANDELIONS	94
	GRAPEFRUIT	104
	LEMONS	112
	LETTUCE	117
	PEANUTS	133
	PRUNES	145
	TURNIPS	167
	WATERCRESS	171
Uric acid, excessive	GRAPES	103
Urination, painful	CARROTS	78
Urinary tract, diseases of	APPLES	60
	LETTUCE	117
	PARSLEY	130
Urine, insufficient flow of	CUCUMBERS	92
Urine, sugar in		19, 22
Vitamin A, need for		14, 25, 40, 44
Vitamin B₁ —see Thiamine		
Vitamin B₂ —see Riboflavin		
Vitamin B₆ —see Pyridoxine		
Vitamin B₁₂		48
Vitamin C		49
Vitamin D		28, 50
Vitamin E		14, 25, 51
Vitamin F		52
Vitamin G		44
Vitamin H (Biotin)		53
Vitamin K		53
Vitamin P		54
Vitamins, need for		39
Voice, hoarseness of	APRICOTS	62
	ASPARAGUS	63
	BARLEY	66
	BEANS	67
	BEET GREENS	70
	BLACK WALNUTS	169
	BRAZIL NUTS	72

Voice *(cont.)*